Elimination Disorders in Children and Adolescents

D1451984

About the Authors

Edward R. Christophersen, PhD, received his doctorate in Developmental and Child Psychology from the University of Kansas in 1970. He is a Fellow in the American Psychological Association and is Board Certified (by examination) in Clinical Psychology by the American Board of Professional Psychology. He has published 10 books (the most notable was *Treatments that Work with Children: Empirically Supported Strategies for Childhood Problems*, a best selling textbook), 181 papers and chapters, and given over 600 presentations at regional and national conferences. He has been the recipient (as PI or Co-PI) of 38 grants with total direct costs of over six million dollars. In recognition of his unique contributions in the area of child health and development, in 1998 he was made an Honorary Fellow in the American Academy of Pediatrics.

Patrick C. Friman, PhD, ABPP is the Director of Clinical Services at Boys Town in Omaha Nebraska and a Clinical Professor of Pediatrics at the University of Nebraska School of Medicine. Dr. Friman is a Fellow in the American Psychological Association and is Board Certified (by examination) in Cognitive and Behavioral Psychology by the American Board of Professional Psychology. He has published two books and more than 170 papers in scientific journals and books. He is the former editor of the *Journal of Applied Behavior Analysis*, is currently on the editorial boards of nine peer reviewed journals, and is the president elect of the Association of Behavior Analysis International.

Advances in Psychotherapy – Evidence-Based Practice

Danny Wedding; PhD, MPH, Prof., St. Louis, MO
(Series Editor)
Larry Beutler; PhD, Prof., Palo Alto, CA
Kenneth E. Freedland; PhD, Prof., St. Louis, MO
Linda C. Sobell; PhD, ABPP, Prof., Ft. Lauderdale, FL
David A. Wolfe; PhD, Prof., Toronto
(Associate Editors)

The basic objective of this series is to provide therapists with practical, evidence-based treatment guidance for the most common disorders seen in clinical practice – and to do so in a "reader-friendly" manner. Each book in the series is both a compact "how-to-do" reference on a particular disorder for use by professional clinicians in their daily work, as well as an ideal educational resource for students and for practice-oriented continuing education.

The most important feature of the books is that they are practical and "reader-friendly:" All are structured similarly and all provide a compact and easy-to-follow guide to all aspects that are relevant in real-life practice. Tables, boxed clinical "pearls", marginal notes, and summary boxes assist orientation, while checklists provide tools for use in daily practice.

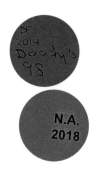

Elimination Disorders in Children and Adolescents

Edward R. Christophersen
University of Missouri at Kansas City School of Medicine and Children's
Mercy Hospital, Kansas City, MO

Patrick C. Friman
Clinical Services at Boys Town in Omaha, NE and the University of
Nebraska School of Medicine

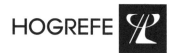

Library of Congress Cataloging in Publication

is available via the Library of Congress Marc Database under the
LC Control Number 2009939400

Library and Archives Canada Cataloguing in Publication

Christophersen, Edward R.
          Elimination disorders in children and adolescents /
Edward R. Christophersen, Patrick C. Friman.

(Advances in psychotherapy--evidence-based practice)
Includes bibliographical references.
ISBN 978-0-88937-334-1

          1. Encopresis. 2. Constipation in children. 3. Enuresis.
I. Friman, Patrick C. II. Title. III. Series: Advances in
psychotherapy--evidence-based practice

RJ456.F43C57 2009   618.92'342   C2009-906408-1

Cover picture: © 2006 Jorge Delgado, available from www.iStockphoto.com

PUBLISHING OFFICES
USA: Hogrefe Publishing, 875 Massachusetts Avenue, 7th Floor, Cambridge, MA 02139
                  Phone (866) 823-4726, Fax (617) 354-6875; E-mail customerservice@hogrefe-publishing.com
EUROPE: Hogrefe Publishing, Rohnsweg 25, 37085 Göttingen, Germany
                  Phone +49 551 49609-0, Fax +49 551 49609-88, E-mail publishing@hogrefe.com

SALES & DISTRIBUTION
USA: Hogrefe Publishing, Customer Services Department,
                  30 Amberwood Parkway, Ashland, OH 44805
                  Phone (800) 228-3749, Fax (419) 281-6883, E-mail customerservice@hogrefe.com
EUROPE: Hogrefe Publishing, Rohnsweg 25, 37085 Göttingen, Germany
                  Phone +49 551 49609-0, Fax +49 551 49609-88, E-mail publishing@hogrefe.com

OTHER OFFICES
CANADA: Hogrefe Publishing, 660 Eglinton Ave. East, Suite 119-514, Toronto, Ontario, M4G 2K2
SWITZERLAND: Hogrefe Publishing, Länggass-Strasse 76, CH-3000 Bern 9

Hogrefe Publishing
Incorporated and registered in the Commonwealth of Massachusetts, USA, and in Göttingen, Lower Saxony,
Germany

Printed and bound in the USA
ISBN: 978-0-88937-334-1

Table of Contents

1

General Introduction

The elimination of bodily waste is a simple mammalian behavior with a multitude of meanings. It can mark territory, project anger, represent fear, initiate play, and even intensify sexual congress. It can also pose problems: Mammalian prey often meet an untimely demise when carnivorous predators track them by attending to the scent of their waste. Not surprisingly, the elimination of bodily waste of humans has generated the most meanings – almost bizarre in its range – and caused the most problems in the mammalian world. It extends from the psychosexual meanings supplied by Freud and his followers to the triad of characteristics (i.e., fire-setting, cruelty to animals, bedwetting) used historically (Hellman & Blackman, 1966) and spuriously (e.g., Slavkin & Shohov, 2004) to identify persons predisposed to violent crime. Human beings seem to enjoy generating complex meaning, even when the subject of their musings involves such simple substances as urine and feces. The range of problems created by the elimination of waste is also very broad, extending from health problems (e.g., infection, compaction, reflux) to social problems (e.g., rejection, ridicule) to family problems (e.g., abuse, neglect) to psychological problems (e.g., anxiety, depression).

As in so many other domains of human life, the scientific approach to the elimination of bodily waste by humans has dramatically simplified and reduced the meanings attributed to it and solved – or at least simplified – almost all the problems it can cause. This book focuses on two of the many problems, namely, childhood encopresis and enuresis. Although many persons have contributed in the past to the scientific progress made in the study of these conditions, each has a scientific patron saint, as it were. For enuresis, Herbert Mowrer was the first and the foremost early investigator to explore the utility of the so-called urine alarm in the treatment of nocturnal enuresis (Mowrer & Mowrer, 1938). For encopresis, Murray Davidson was the first and the foremost early investigator to explore the utility of stool softeners in the treatment of encopresis (Davidson, 1958). In so doing, both individuals inaugurated lines of investigation that gradually grew, elbowed out arcane, speculative and nonproductive perspectives on enuresis and encopresis, and eventually resulted in the empirically supported biobehavioral approaches to assessment and treatment used today.

In this book we cover each condition comprehensively in a specified sequence: multicomponent descriptions (e.g., definition, diagnosis, epidemiology, etc.), influential theories and models, major approaches to treatment, problems encountered carrying out treatments, and case vignettes. The book is divided into three sections: The first covers constipation and encopresis, the second nocturnal enuresis, and the third diurnal enuresis. The encopresis section also includes a discussion on toileting refusal. Consistent with the theme of the series of which this book is a part, we will strongly emphasize and favor evidence-based perspectives on all aspects of both conditions, particularly treatment.

2

Constipation and Encopresis

2.1   Description

2.1.1   Terminology and Definition

Encopresis is the involuntary loss of formed, semiformed, or liquid stool in inappropriate places such as underwear, diapers, or pull-ups in children over 4 years of age (Loening-Baucke, 1996). Primary or continuous encopresis applies to children who have been incontinent their entire lives; secondary or discontinuous encopresis applies to children who were fully bowel-trained at some point (Levine, 1975) and then later resumed soiling. The diagnostic criteria for encopresis, as indicated in the *Diagnostic and Statistical Manual of Mental Disorders*, Fourth Edition (DSM-IV; American Psychiatric Association, 1994), may be found in Table 1.

> **Primary or continuous encopresis applies to children who have been incontinent their entire lives**

Other terminology important to the understanding of encopresis are *Hirschsprung disease, constipation, and toileting refusal*. Hirschsprung disease (congenital aganglionic megacolon) is a congenital anomaly wherein the furthest part of the child's large intestine lacks appropriate innervation (Christophersen & Mortweet, 2001). Some 40% of children with Hirschsprung disease are diagnosed in the first 3 months, 61% by 12 months, and 82% by 4 years of age (Loening-Baucke, 1994). Hirschsprung disease in the older child causes chronic constipation and abdominal distention. The stools, when

> **Generally, a physician has already ruled out Hirschsprung disease prior to a child being seen by a mental health clinician**

Table 1
DSM-IV Criteria for Encopresis

A. Repeated passage of feces into inappropriate places (e.g., clothing or floor) whether involuntary or intentional.
B. At least one such event a month for at least 3 months.
C. Chronological age is at least 4 years (or equivalent developmental level).
D. The behavior is not due exclusively to the direct physiological effects of a substance (e.g., laxatives) or a general medical condition except through a mechanism involving constipation.

Code as follows:

797.6 With Constipation and Overflow Incontinence: there is evidence of constipation on physical exam or by history

307.7 Without Constipation and Overflow Incontinence: there is no evidence of constipation on physical exam or by history

Reprinted with permission from the *Diagnostic and Statistical Manual of Mental Disorders, Fourth Edition* (© 1994) American Psychiatric Association.

passed, may consist of small pellets, be ribbon-like, or have a fluid consistency; the large stools and fecal soiling of patients with functional constipation are absent. In the vast majority of cases, a physician has already ruled out Hirschsprung disease prior to a child being seen by a clinician (Christophersen & Mortweet, 2001). Further information on distinguishing Hirschsprung disease from encopresis may be found in the "Differential Diagnosis and Diagnostic Procedures and Documentation" discussions of this section of the book.

Constipation has been defined as the passage of large or hard stools at a frequency of less than 3 times per week (Sutphen, Borowitz, Hutchison, & Cox, 1995). Luxem and Christophersen (1999) defined constipation as "hard stools that are difficult to pass," rather than referring to the frequency of stooling. They also reported that constipation in children may be accompanied by complaints of abdominal discomfort, infrequent bowel movements (e.g., fewer than three bowel movements a week), a palpable abdominal mass, emotional upset, including crying and screaming before, during, and after defecation, vigorous attempts at bowel-movement withholding, nausea and vomiting, poor appetite, weight loss, sadness and irritability, and leaking of small amounts of stools which the children often report not feeling. Occasionally, children with encopresis (secondary to constipation) are able to pass enough feces to plug up toilets. A history of constipation in one or both parents may also predispose a child to constipation as a result of an abnormally long colonic transit time, overly efficient intestinal absorption of water, or both. Schonwald and Sheldon (2006) stated that "constipation doesn't mean that the child hardly ever poops; it means that the poops often hurt or are hard to make."

> **"Toileting refusal" refers to children who refuse to have a bowel movement in the toilet but will use a diaper or a pull-up**

Toileting refusal is used to refer to children who refuse to have a bowel movement in the toilet but who willingly have a bowel movement in a diaper or a pull-up (Luxem, Christophersen, Purvis, & Baer, 1997). Toileting refusal is discussed in a separate section below. Children with encopresis may come to the attention of the clinician through a referral from the child's physician for assistance with bowel retraining, or while obtaining the history via a diagnostic interview for a different problem. The differential diagnosis of these toileting disorders are outlined in more detail later in the book.

2.1.2   Epidemiology

2.1.2.1   Prevalence

> **The prevalence of encopresis in the US ranges from 1% to 3%, affecting boys 3–6 times more often than girls**

Schonwald and Rappaport (2008) estimated that the prevalence of encopresis in the United States ranges from 1% to 3%, affecting boys 3–6 times more often than girls. Levine (1975) reported a slightly higher prevalence rate of clinic-referred cases at 3%. Levine also reported that the mean age of onset for secondary encopresis is 7 years and 4 months of age. Despite the prevalence of encopresis, it has been called a "hidden disease" in at least one published report (Brody, 1992). Parents of children with encopresis often think that they are the *only* family who has a child with this problem (Christophersen & Mortweet, 2001). In addition, the fact that encopresis is rarely mentioned in the popular press may contribute to this misconception. Clearly, there are other medical conditions with an incidence rate of far less than 1%–3% that are mentioned more regularly than encopresis in the media. For example, in children under 20 years of age in the United States the incidence of diabetes is less than 1%.

Since constipation is often directly related to encopresis, it is important to report the prevalence rates for constipation as well. More than 90% of children referred for the treatment of encopresis present with functional constipation (Schonwald & Rappaport, 2008). The prevalence of constipation – and thus, possibly encopresis – appears to be increasing, although no apparent explanation has been reported in the literature for this increase (Christophersen & Mortweet, 2001).

2.1.3 Etiology

Although numerous theories have been offered on the etiology of encopresis, including coercive toilet training, a history of hostile or violent events, and child abuse, the only etiological factor we could find support for in the literature was constipation. Constipation plays a major role in encopresis as well as in other toileting problems such as withholding, which can create and exacerbate stooling difficulties. In fact, constipation-related problems, including encopresis and toileting refusal are usually present in children who are referred to gastroenterology clinics (Luxem et al., 1997).

The fecal elimination process is profoundly affected by diet and behavior. The motility of the colon is easily reduced either involuntarily, due to insufficient bulk or roughage or too many bland foods in the diet, or voluntarily due to toileting refusal. Reduced motility results in excess quantities of moisture being drawn off the fecal mass making it dryer than normal and thus reducing colonic motility even further. This pattern can lead to a regressive cycle in which the retention of feces decreases motility – leading to further retention of feces. This cycle then becomes a primary cause of constipation and fecal incontinence. Not surprisingly, the vast majority of children with encopresis have histories of constipation (Friman & Jones, 1998; Levine, 1982).

Precisely establishing the etiology for this constipation/soiling cycle is a difficult assignment. However, there are several behavioral/dietary factors with a known causative role. These include (1) insufficient roughage or bulk; (2) a bland diet, too high in dairy products and cheeses, resulting in reduced colonic motility; (3) insufficient oral intake of fluids (which allows the normal reabsorption of water from the colon to dehydrate the feces too much) or dehydration stemming from activities that increase the loss of fluids by sweating; (4) fecal retention by the child; (5) medications that have the side effect of promoting constipation (such as drugs that are used to control seizures or attention deficit hyperactivity disorder, and narcotics used to control pain); and (6) the child's emotional state. Any of these factors, singly or in combination, can result in constipation-like symptoms or actual constipation. Loening-Baucke, Cruikshank, and Savage (1987) found that the persistence of encopresis at 6-month and 12-month follow-ups was not related to social competence, but was significantly related to the inability to defecate and relax the external anal sphincter during defecation attempts.

When a child with a history of uncomfortable or painful bowel movements feels the urge to defecate, he or she may associate that urge with sensations that occurred previously and were followed by a painful or uncomfortable bowel movement. In an attempt to prevent a recurrence of the painful bowel movement, the child may then voluntarily retain feces, thus exacerbating the problem. If constipation is extended, the child may become lethargic, which in turn reduces activity levels, the reduced activity leads to an additional decrease in colonic motility, the constipation is perpetuated and so on. More severe constipation may also result in a decreased appetite. The child may develop a fecal impaction or a large blockage caused by the collection of hard dry stool. Not infrequently, these children experience seepage around the fecal mass, producing what has been termed "paradoxical diarrhea" (Levine, 1982): Although the child is actually constipated, he or she appears to have diarrhea. Some parents may even attempt to treat this type of "diarrhea" with over-the counter antidiarrheal agents that only worsen the problem.

2.1.4   Course and Prognosis

As with other childhood disorders, a thorough history of the child's and the family's physical and mental health should be obtained. This history should include questions about the family medical history, the child's stooling habits, the child's diet history, and information about any previous attempts to deal with the encopresis, including rewards or punishment. Healthcare providers may find that having parents complete a detailed history prior to the child's first appointment can increase the efficiency of the initial intake interview.

Relief from constipation can be accomplished by administering medications orally or rectally.

There are two often distinct goals in the treatment of encopresis. If the child is constipated or impacted, the first goal is to relieve the constipation or impaction (Christophersen & Mortweet, 2001), which can be accomplished by administering medications orally or rectally. There are no outcome-based studies comparing the efficacy of these two routes of administration. As Stark (2000) stated, the specific regimen for a bowel cleanout can vary and includes enemas, suppositories, and large doses of mineral oil or a balanced electrolyte lavage solution given by mouth or nasogastric tube. One argument that has been made for the use of oral methods of bowel cleanout is that enemas may be "psychologically unsuitable." However, there is little empirical data to support such an assertion; some survey data indicate that, although children find enemas difficult, over half of the children treated with this modality reported enemas to be useful (p. 255–256).

In the absence of empirical data to help one decide which route to take, we often rely on the decision of the primary care provider. In extreme cases we refer to a pediatric gastroenterologist to relieve the constipation or clean out the colon. In our experience, practitioners new to this area may sometimes come close to apologizing to parents for the need for an initial cleanout, which reflects a lack of understanding of why such as cleanout is so necessary. Without an adequate cleanout, progress may be quite limited. In some cases, we take the approach of getting the child started on a diet that is higher in dietary fiber and lower in milk and other dairy products at least several days prior to the cleanout, which frequently gives much better results.

The second goal, after the child's colon has been cleaned out, is to implement a treatment regimen that will keep the child from getting constipated again. Although the initial cleanout is usually done within a couple of days at most, it may take months for the muscle in the intestine to heal. During this time, it is important to offer whatever incentives may be necessary to maintain the child's cooperation with the treatment regimen. These strategies are discussed in detail later in this book.

2.1.5 Differential Diagnosis

"For most children with encopresis, assessment can be limited to the history and physical examination alone" (Schonwald & Rapport, 2008, p. 797). Yet getting a good history requires the examiner be familiar with normal toileting practices to ascertain when a toileting history is in fact remarkable.

Although many pediatric textbooks recommend a digital rectal examination (DRE) by a physician to assess for constipation and impaction (cf. Schonwald & Rappaport, 2008), the procedure is not performed in the majority of children evaluated for chronic constipation. Safder, Rewalt, and Elitsur (2006), in a review of the literature on DRE in children with constipation, stated that primary-care physicians "only rarely perform this examination" (p. 411). DRE was performed by the referring physician in only 15% of the patients, compared to 96% by the specialist. The DRE, when performed by an experienced practitioner, is a very useful component in the evaluation of a child presenting with constipation (Rockney, McQuade, & Days, 1995).

Negative findings of constipation at the time of physical examination do not necessarily rule out constipation, because evidence of constipation may be only intermittent (Christophersen & Mortweet, 2001). In cases in which the history is consistent with constipation (but constipation cannot be confirmed by the physical examination), a plain X-ray of the abdomen may be necessary (Levine, 1982). Barr, Levine, Wilkinson, and Mulvihill (1979) used X-rays to assess the degree of retention and reported significant differences between pre- and posttherapy X-rays of treatment successes, but no differences between pre- and posttherapy X-rays of treatment failures. Rockney et al. (1995) used plain X-ray films – an objective, reliable, assessment tool – to film the abdomens of 60 children with encopresis and documented that 78% of the children had fecal retention. Using the plain film of the abdomen as the gold standard, a rectal examination showed a positive predictive value of 85% and a negative predictive value of 50% in assessing fecal retention. These findings lend further support to the notion that the vast majority of children with encopresis have physical findings related to their colon that should be reviewed by the child's physician.

It is important to rule out Hirschsprung disease as a cause. Hirschsprung disease, or congenital aganglionic megacolon, involves an enlargement of the colon caused by bowel obstruction resulting from an aganglionic section of bowel (the normal enteric nerves being absent) that starts at the anus and progresses upwards. Levine (1983) provided a list (Table 2) of the common symptoms of Hirschsprung disease and encopresis in a format that can be readily incorporated into the clinical interview for a child who presents with encopresis. There are several symptoms (e.g., late onset, problems with toilet training, and stool incontinence) common among children with encopresis but rare in children with Hirschsprung disease, and there are symptoms that are common

Table 2
Symptoms of Encopresis and Hirschsprung Disease

Characteristic	Encopresis	Hirschsprung Disease
Stool incontinence	Always	Rare
Constipation	Common, may be intermittent	Always
Symptoms as newborn	Rare	Almost always
Infant constipation	Sometimes	Common
Late onset (after age 3)	Common	Rare
Problem toilet training	Common	Rare
Avoidance of toilet	Common	Rare
Failure to Thrive	Rare	Common
Anemia	None	Common
Obstructive symptoms	Rare	Common
Stool in ampulla	Common	Rare
Loose or tight sphincter tone	Rare	Common
Large caliber stools	Common	Never
Preponderance of males	86%	90%
Incidence	1.5% at age 7	1:25,000 births
Anal manometry	Sometimes abnormal	Always abnormal

Adapted from Levine, M.D. (1983). Encopresis. In M.D. Levine, W.B. Carey, & A.C. Crocker (Eds.), *Developmental-behavioral pediatrics* (2nd ed., pp. 389-397). Philadelphia: Saunders. Reprinted with permission.

among children with Hirschsprung disease but rare in children with encopresis (e.g., failure to thrive, anemia). Symptoms for Hirschsprung disease are rarely, if ever, seen in children with either encopresis or toileting refusal.

2.1.6   Comorbidities

The most common comorbidity in children with encopresis is constipation

The most common comorbidity in children with encopresis is constipation. Partin, Hamill, Fischel, and Partin (1992), in a study of over 200 children who presented with encopresis at a gastroenterology clinic, reported that 85% of the children also suffered from stool withholding, fecal impaction, and pain on defecation. Of the children older than 3 years, 96% exhibited stool withholding, 57% had painful defecation, 73% showed fecal impaction, and 85% presented with encopresis. They also reported that, of the children under 3 years of age, over 70% had fecal impaction and painful defecation, suggesting that they also had problems with constipation. The majority of these children (71%) also suffered from fecal impaction, a condition in which the colon is so full of stool that peristalsis is inhibited.

2.1.7 Diagnostic Procedures and Documentation

2.1.7.1 Medical Assessment

If a child has been referred for treatment by a pediatrician, the first thing to do is establish how much evaluation has already been done. We have had children referred who had absolutely no evaluation (i.e., the parent asked about getting treatment for their child's encopresis and the pediatrician referred them on); and we have had children referred by board-certified pediatric gastroenterologists only after an extensive workup and a medication trial with MiraLax™. Practicing in a large children's hospital (ERC) is an obvious advantage, because any prior evaluation is usually present in the child's medical record.

> If a child has been referred for treatment by a pediatrician, first establish how much evaluation has already been done

2.1.7.2 Evaluation

Our rule of "go no further with treatment until the child has received a medical evaluation" is important for all elimination problems discussed in this book, but it may be most important for encopresis. Apart from the possibility of organic disease (discussed below), there is still the very serious problem of excessive waste accumulating in an organ with a finite amount of space. Unfortunately, an all too frequent problem in medical clinics is when an encopretic child presents who had been in extended therapy with a nonmedical professional, whose initial evaluation did not include referral for a medical evaluation, and whose treatment did not address known causes of encopresis (e.g., diet, behavior, constipation). The child's colonic system can become painfully and dangerously distended – sometimes to the point of being life threatening (e.g., McGuire, Rothenberg, & Tyler, 1983).

> Our rule of "go no further with treatment until the child has received a medical evaluation" is important for all elimination problems, especially encopresis

Regardless of prior treatments, a thorough history of the child's stooling habits since infancy should be obtained. In their more classical presentation, constipation and difficult stooling often start when the parent introduces formula to a child who has previously been breastfed. We find it interesting that pear juice, which is frequently recommended for constipation because it helps to keep stools soft and moist, is usually sold in the infant section of grocery stores, rather than in either the juice or the pharmacy sections. Clearly, store managers know that pear juice, properly placed in the infant section, sells.

To treat encopresis effectively, special attention should be paid to any evidence of prior or current constipation in the child's history (Christophersen & Mortweet, 2001). The Society for Pediatric Gastroenterology, and Nutrition, in its *Clinical Practice Guidelines on the Evaluation and Treatment of Constipation* (2006), defines constipation as "a delay or difficulty in defecation, present for two or more weeks."

Such historical information should include stooling frequency, stool size, stool consistency, any prior problems such as bleeding, and any prior interventions attempted by professionals or by the parents using home remedies (Christophersen & Mortweet, 2001). Many parents fail to recognize constipation in their child, apparently assuming that as long as the child has a bowel movement on most days, he or she "couldn't have constipation." In fact, children can indeed have daily bowel movements and still be constipated. The child, who is having daily bowel movements but not actually expelling all of the waste matter from the rectum, can gradually accumulate larger and larger amounts of fecal matter (Christophersen, 1994). Also, although some children

Table 3
DSM-IV Differential

Toileting refusal	Encopresis 307.7	Hirschsprung disease
• Regular stools	• Repeated soilings	• Anemia as an infant
• Never in toilet	• at least 1/month	• Easy to toilet train
• In diaper/pull-ups	• Not physiological	• Failure to thrive
• Age 3 or over	• Age 4 or over	• Family history of colon Dx
• Hx of constipation	• Hx of constipation	
_____ of 5 (4+ = Dx)	_____ of 5 (4+ = Dx)	_____ of 4 (3+ = Dx)

defecate only every 3–5 days, their parents might assume that they are not constipated because they have bowel accidents; and on the days without any bowel accidents, their children used the toilet appropriately. In school-age children, soiling accidents tend to occur at home, typically after school between 3 and 7 p.m. (Levine, 1976), although children with a history of chronic and frequent soiling may have accidents outside the home and at various times throughout the day. Only rarely do children soil during their sleep. Parents report that their children are often observed to be standing upright, walking or engaged in vigorous play when soiling occurs (Luxem & Christophersen, 1999).

It is rare for children to soil during their sleep

A number of medications, such as pain medications and some anticonvulsants, relax the intestine and may produce or aggravate constipation as a side effect. For this reason, asking parents to complete a detailed history form and bring it with them to the first office visit helps identify any medication-related constipation problems. Also, because some parents mistake "overflow" diarrhea for actual diarrhea, children who soil may also have been treated by their parents, with the best of intentions, with antidiarrheal medications such as Imodium™, Pepto-Bismol™, or a number of over-the-counter or prescription medications for diarrhea.

A number of medications may produce or aggravate constipation as a side effect

In the authors' experience, in the vast majority of cases a primary-care physician has already ruled out Hirschsprung disease prior to the child being seen by a mental-health practitioner. If a primary-care physician has not seen a child, such a referral is indicated. To facilitate a differential diagnosis of encopresis, Table 3 provides a list of the symptoms of toileting refusal, encopresis, and Hirschsprung disease. Although toileting refusal and Hirschsprung disease are not included in DSM-IV (American Psychiatric Association, 1994), these conditions must be ruled out as part of the diagnosis of encopresis.

2.1.7.3 Behavioral Assessment

Assessment of the child's history of toilet-training should include a review of the onset and duration of the child's bowel and bladder training, the methods used, and the behavioral responses of the child, parents, and other persons involved in the training process (Luxem & Christophersen, 1999). Evaluation of previous treatments for the child's constipation and soiling, including behavioral and psychological interventions, can reveal telling evidence of the ability and willingness of the child and the child's parents to adhere to treatment recommendations. For example, parents commonly report that their child "hides soiled underwear" (Schonwald & Sheldon, 2006), which suggests a prior history of punishment for soiling. When there is such a history, it is imperative that the parents be thoroughly educated about the most common causes of encopresis, so they understand that the child is not soiling intentionally, and that punishment for soiling is rarely effective (Christophersen & Mortweet, 2001).

Although most early studies documented the absence of significant behavior problems in children with encopresis (Friman, Mathews, Christophersen, & Leibowitz, 1988; Gabel, Hegedus, Wald, Chandra, & Chiponis, 1986), more recent studies have suggested that children with encopresis do present with more psychological problems than children without encopresis (Cox, Morris, Borowitz, & Sutphen, 2002; Joinson, Heron, Butler, & von Gontard, 2006). Cox et al. (2002) compared 86 children with encopresis to 62 nonsymptomatic children on five psychometric instruments (Child Behavior Checklist, CBCL Teacher Report Form, Family Environmental Scale, Wide Range Achievement Test – Revised, and Piers-Harris). They reported that, as a group, children with encopresis differ from children without encopresis on a variety of psychological parameters, but that only a minority of children with encopresis demonstrated clinically significant elevations in these parameters. Joinson et al. (2006) conducted a population-based study on a total of 8,242 children aged 7–8 years and born to mothers in the United Kingdom. They compared children who soil frequently with children who soil occasionally and children who do not soil at all:

"Children who soil were reported by their parents to have significantly more emotional and behavioral problems compared with children who do not soil (p. 1575)."

However, whether soiling caused emotional and behavioral problems or vice versa cannot be answered based upon their reported data.

In our opinion, both parents and teachers should be asked to complete a standardized rating scale such as the Child Behavior Checklist (CBCL; Achenbach, 1991) or the Behavior Assessment System for Children (BASC; Reynolds & Kamphaus, 1992) to ascertain – prior to any treatment attempt – that the child does or does not present with significant behavior problems. If the history and the rating scales are significant for behavior problems, the treatment of encopresis may be more complicated. The clinician must then decide whether first to treat the encopresis or the problems with behavior management. Christophersen (1994) suggests that this determination can be made based upon whether the history and rating scales document significant problems with behaviors, such as defiance and difficulty following instructions. These behavior problems may interfere with the parents' or the child's ability to adhere to the treatment recommendations. If adherence has been or is expected to be a problem, Christophersen (1994) recommends introducing small changes such as a slight modification of the diet (described later in this chapter) and then concentrating on dealing with the adherence issues.

Both parents and teachers should be asked to complete a standardized rating scale to assess behavorial problems

Prior to Davidson's (1958) seminal work on constipation and encopresis, the common misconception was that encopresis was a symptom of an underlying mental health problem (Richmond, Eddy, & Garrard, 1954). Mellon, Whiteside, and Friedrich (2006) addressed the issue of soiling as an indicator of sexual abuse by comparing 466 children referred and treated for sexual abuse with 429 psychiatrically referred children and 641 normative children

The predictive utility of fecal soiling as an indicator of sexual abuse is not supported by research

recruited from the community. They concluded that the "predictive utility of fecal soiling as an indicator of sexual abuse is not supported" (p. 25).

2.2   Theories and Models of Constipation and Encopresis

2.2.1   Physiological Factors

The large intestine or colon is the distal end of the alimentary tract, sequentially composed of the esophagus, stomach, biliary tract, and the intestines (small and large). The colon has three major functions: storage of waste, fluid absorption from waste, and evacuation of waste. Extended storage and planned evacuation of fecal waste into an appropriate location are the defining features of fecal continence. Evacuation is achieved through a motor function called peristalsis, which involves a wavelike motion of the walls of the colon. Retrograde peristalsis in the ascending colon keeps liquid fecal waste in contact with the absorptive walls of the colon, resulting in gradual solidification of the waste, which begins to move forward as it takes on mass. Movement occurs over an extended period and is potentiated by external events, for example, gross motor activity (resulting in the orthocolic reflex) and eating (resulting in the gastrocolic reflex).

The rectum usually contains little or no fecal matter. But when colonic movement leads to the contraction of the sigmoid colon, feces are propelled into the rectum and its distension stimulates sensory receptors in the rectal mucosa and in the muscles of the pelvic floor. Two muscle-based "switching systems" – the internal and external sphincters – regulate fecal progression from that point. The internal sphincter is involuntary and opens only through the stimulation generated by the process described above. As fecal mass distends the rectum, the child can manipulate the external sphincter using three muscle groups (thoracic diaphragm, abdominal musculature, and *levator ani*) to start or stop defecation. (These muscle groups are also used to start or stop urination – described more fully in the enuresis section.) Thus, as with the achievement of urinary continence, fecal continence requires appropriate responses to stimulation generated by a waste-receiving organ system. In very general terms, the purpose of fecal toilet training is to acquaint the child with the proprioceptive feedback from the colon and to coordinate the relaxing of the external anal sphincter with sitting on a toilet (Friman & Jones, 1998; Weinstock & Clouse, 1987)

Encopresis was once thought to be a psychiatric disorder (Richmond et al., 1954). Davidson (1958) was one of the first authors to challenge the long-standing notion that the cause was psychogenic. Davidson's work was also instrumental in recognizing the important role that constipation plays in the etiology of encopresis. His treatment program focused on managing the child's constipation first and toilet training second. His program has been labeled the "pediatric approach"; it relied primarily on the use of mineral oil to treat the child's constipation.

Borowitz et al. (2003) compared symptoms that occurred during the 3 months before a child presented with a chief complaint of constipation at a primary-care physician's office to children without a history of constipation (including both nonconstipated siblings and nonsiblings). They reported that painful defecation was the primary precipitant of constipation during early childhood. Parents of constipated children indicated that their children had more difficult and more painful defecation experiences than did the control children, and the constipated children were more likely to express worry about future defecation than were the control children. Painful defecation was by far the event most commonly reported before the onset of constipation as well as the event most often described as causing constipation.

In addition to suffering from constipation, children with encopresis may have a diminished sensation in their rectum are thus less likely to perceive the "call to stool" needed for appropriate elimination (Christophersen & Mortweet, 2001). For example, Meunier, Mollard, and Marechal (1976) used anal manometry to determine the rectum sensitivity of children with and without normal bowel histories. They established a laboratory procedure in which a small tube was inserted into the patient's rectum. One or more portions of the tube could then be inflated until the patients subjectively reported feeling as though they were about to have a bowel movement. The amount of pressure necessary to create that feeling was duly noted. This procedure allowed the researchers to simulate the increased pressure in the rectum that an individual normally feels prior to having a bowel movement. In the Meunier et al. study, most of the children with normal bowel histories required only a small amount of pressure in the rectum, whereas most of the children with encopresis required 2–4 times as much pressure before they felt the "call to stool." The data presented here lend support to the comment often heard from children with encopresis that they "couldn't feel the bowel movement coming."

> Children with encopresis may have diminished sensation in their rectum so that they are less likely to perceive the "call to stool"

Further support for the role of biological factors in encopresis was provided by Ingebo and Heyman (1988), who conducted a study to determine whether children with encopresis retained more stool in their rectum than did children without encopresis. They conducted a clinical trial using an oral solution, GoLytely (polyethylene-glycol-electrolyte), with 24 children, ages 9 months to 17 years, with severe constipation (Christophersen & Mortweet, 2001). Approximately 50% of the children were being treated for encopresis, while the other half were being prepared for colonoscopy. The children with encopresis required almost 3 times as much medication, administered over 3 times as long a period of time, in order to clean out the colon. These results support the notion that children with encopresis retain more stool and require more medication over a longer period of time than do children not presenting with encopresis. The author reported no clinically important changes in the laboratory values measured before and after the intestinal cleanout in either group of children, suggesting that the use of enemas to "clean out" the colon is not detrimental to children.

2.2.2   Psychiatric Factors

For many years, encopresis was viewed as a psychiatric disorder or symptom of emotional disturbance. A number of studies specifically examined the notion that children with encopresis have emotional or behavioral problems.

The use of child-behavior rating scales, such as the Achenbach Child Behavior Checklist (Achenbach, 1991), revealed no systematic differences between children with encopresis and normal children of the same age and gender (Christophersen & Mortweet, 2001). Rating scales also showed that children with encopresis tend to be more well adjusted than same-age, same-sex samples of children with "behavior problems" (Gabel et al., 1986; Loening-Baucke et al., 1987). Friman et al. (1988) reported that children referred for management of encopresis did not differ significantly from the standardization sample for the Eyberg Child Behavior Inventory (Robinson, Eyberg, & Ross, 1980). Further, both the children with encopresis and the standardization sample differed significantly from children who were referred for diagnosis and management of behavior problems.

Loening-Baucke et al. (1987) examined the social competence and behavioral profiles of 38 children with encopresis, with a specific interest in children resistant to treatment. They concluded that the persistence of encopresis at 6-month and 12-month follow-ups after the initiation of treatment was not related to social competence or to behavior scores. Given the existence of research that clearly demonstrates the presence of significant physical findings and the absence of research demonstrating consistent behavior problems in the vast majority of children diagnosed and treated for encopresis, we propose that encopresis can and should be treated primarily as a dysfunction of the bowel.

Schonwald, Sherritt, Stadtler, and Bridgemohan (2004) compared 46 children referred for difficult toilet training with 62 comparison children, using three measures of temperament. They reported that difficult toilet training is associated with difficult temperament and constipation. They reported no differences in parenting styles. Interestingly, they noted that 55% of the children in the comparison group had histories of constipation compared to 78% of the children referred for difficult toilet training, leading the authors to conclude that constipation is very common in this age group. Their results were based on a "toileting history questionnaire" that is currently not in the public domain and thus not available for inspection. If this study were replicated, temperament could be added to the list of factors that contribute to difficult toilet training.

2.3   Treatment for Constipation and Encopresis

A first step in treating encopresis is to ensure that parents understand that their child is most likely *not* soiling on purpose

After an initial assessment to ascertain the extent to which a child with encopresis also presents with behavioral or emotional problems, most authors seem to agree that the first step in treating encopresis is to ensure that parents understand that, in all likelihood, their child is *not* soiling on purpose, and that the child may not have control over his or her soiling.

2.3.1   Providing Education

Ever since Levine introduced the educational procedure he referred to as "demystification" into the literature in 1982, we have been using this pro-

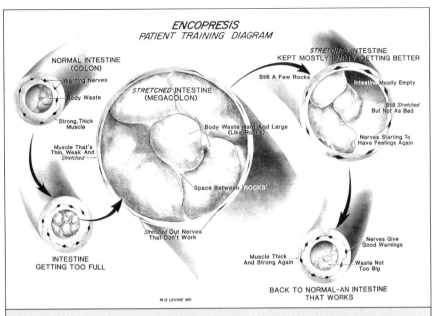

Figure 1
Schematic representation of an normal colon and a megacolon (Reprinted with permission from Levine, 1982, p. 326)

cedure with the vast majority of new referrals of children with encopresis (Levine, 1982). Levine reported that parents often benefited from viewing a simple diagram explaining how abnormal bowel function, in the form of encopresis, can lead to the child's colon being stretched such that they have diminished sensation when they need to have a bowel movement. He made the point that it was important that both parents and child be told that the child was *not* to blame for his or her abnormal bowel functioning, and that effective treatment methods are available (Christophersen & Mortweet, 2001).

Figure 1 is the diagram used by Levine (1982) to help parents understand that their child's bowel "problem" is not intentional soiling. Clinicians can use this diagram to explain to both the child and the parents what factors are present in encopresis, including "the muscles that are thin, weak, and stretched" (i.e., the majority of children with encopresis have a larger diameter rectum than children without encopresis) as well as "warning nerves that don't work" (i.e., children with encopresis often report – correctly – that they cannot feel the "call to stool").

Both parents and child should be told that the child is not to blame for his or her encopresis, and that effective treatment is available

2.3.1.1 Relieving Constipation
After explaining the mechanics of encopresis to the child and parents, the clinician can then introduce the steps for successful treatment. The first step is to reduce or eliminate the large amounts of stool that many of these children have retained in their colon, often referred to as "cleaning out the colon" (Christophersen & Mortweet, 2001). Families can be told that, in order to help the muscles "heal," one must first make sure that the intestine or colon is completely empty.

The first treatment step is to reduce or eliminate the large amounts of stool retained in the colon

The most common way to effectively clean out the child's colon, based on the individual works of Davidson and Levine, is the use of at least one enema. Since no studies exist comparing the oral route (stool softeners, laxatives, or lubricants) with the rectal route (enemas or suppositories) for relieving constipation, we recommend discussing treatment options with the child and parents. This step in encopresis management is vital: If a child with constipation is not adequately cleaned out, neither the constipation nor the encopresis is likely to resolve. For this reason, we routinely recommend that the clinician be quite thorough. So, initially, when deciding between 1 ml/kg or 2 ml/kg of mineral oil or 17 grams of MiraLax™, it is probably better to use too much rather than too little. For those practitioners who are not trained in these procedures, referral back to the primary-care physician may be necessary. And in those cases in which the primary-care physician is not comfortable handling the "cleanout," referral to a pediatric gastroenterologist may be indicated.

2.3.1.2   Helping the Child Prevent Further Constipation

Once the child's colon has successfully been cleaned out, the next step is to keep it from getting too full again

Once the child's colon has successfully been cleaned out, the next step is to keep it from getting too full again. There are several components to this step, which can be implemented simultaneously: scheduled toilet sits, oral medications, and suppositories (Christophersen & Mortweet, 2001).

Scheduled toilet sits

The simplest component is a scheduled toilet sit. The child is asked to sit on the toilet for approximately 5 minutes, 2 or 3 times a day, to facilitate good bowel habits. Many children will have a pattern to their soiling and bowel movements, and the toilet sits should be structured around these times. For example, if the child typically soils after school but before dinner, a toilet sit should be scheduled for right after school to train the child's body to eliminate into the toilet at that time. Adherence to these toilet sits can be enhanced by allowing the child to have a special toy or book that can be played with only during toilet sits. Tangible reinforcers for cooperation, such as stickers or special time with a caregiver, can also be helpful. In the experience of the authors, it is of little use to coerce children to do their "toilet sits" at times when they are very unlikely to have a bowel movement. Therefore, the idea of having three toilet sits a day, one after each meal, is usually not necessary. Three toilet sits a day can be justified only for children who have regular bowel movements or bowel accidents in the morning, afternoon, and evening. In our experience, children who have accidents this often usually need to be cleaned out again.

The child's physician can offer recommendations on the use of oral medications

Normally, the child's physician should be able to offer recommendations to the parents on the use of oral medications. The interested practitioner is referred to Baker et al. (1999) for a thorough discussion of the oral medications and dosing that are available in the evidence-based medicine literature for the treatment of constipation.

The most popular current medical treatment for constipation is MiraLax™

Probably the most popular current treatment for constipation is MiraLax™ (polyethylene glycol or PEG). Several recent studies have examined the efficacy and tolerability of MiraLax™, a powder mixed with a liquid. Pashankar, Loening-Bauche, and Bishop (2003) assessed the clinical and biochemical safety profile of therapy with MiraLax™ with 83 children (54 with chronic constipation and 39 with constipation and encopresis), receiving PEG therapy for more than 3 months. At the time of publication, with a mean duration of 8.7 months of treatment, there were no major clinical adverse effects, all children preferring PEG to previously used laxatives. Daily compliance was measured as good in 90% of children.

One of the earliest studies on the behavioral treatment of encopresis (Wright & Walker, 1976) used a combination of behavioral treatment and medical management by recommending the daily use of rectal suppositories and enemas in the event that the child did not have a bowel movement each day.

Numerous authors, including the present authors, reported favorable outcome data with the use of rectal suppositories as one of the treatment components (O'Brien, Ross, & Christophersen, 1986). Wright and Walker (1976) recommended that parents administer one adult glycerine suppository if a certain amount of stool has not been passed for the day. These were then gradually reduced when the child had daily bowel movements.

2.3.1.3   The Role of Diet and Exercise

Perhaps one of the most important and most difficult components of the treatment protocol for encopresis are the lifestyle changes required in diet and exercise. The American Academy of Pediatrics recommends a daily intake of dietary fiber equivalent to the child's age plus five in grams; for example, a 5-year-old child should be eating 10 grams of dietary fiber (5 + 5) per day (Dwyer, 1995). Since most parents do not know how to estimate the amount of dietary fiber their children eat, parents should be provided with written fiber content information (see Appendix 1) to assist them in preparing meals that have adequate amounts of fiber in them.

> **Lifestyle changes in diet and exercise regimens required in encopresis treatment are both important and difficult**

Houts, Mellon, and Whelan (1988) reported on the use of "fiber points" to encourage children with encopresis to increase their intake of dietary fiber. Children were given a list of various foods and their fiber content, with fiber intake (and water intake) being publicly posted on a bar chart. Houts et al. reported a clear increase in appropriate toileting and a decrease in toileting accidents which was maintained at the 1-year follow-up. Because the children increased their intake of dietary fiber, they no longer needed rectal suppositories to maintain appropriate toileting.

We could not locate any studies that examined whether or not commercially available fiber supplements were worse than, equal to, or better than eating high-fiber foods. In our own clinical experience, it does not seem to matter much what the child is eating as long as he/she is getting an adequate intake of dietary fiber. Another issue that has not been satisfactorily addressed in the literature is the comparison between soluble and insoluble fiber. Apple sauce is an example of a soluble fiber, corn on the cob an example of an insoluble fiber. We usually recommend that parents emphasize the importance of eating insoluble fiber because it seems to promote gastric motility better than soluble fiber. However, this recommendation awaits empirical support.

> **No data exist documenting whether commercially available fiber supplements are worse than, equal to, or better than eating high-fiber foods**

Changes in dairy consumption may also be required for treatment. Davidson (1958), in addition to identifying constipation as a primary etiological factor in pediatric encopresis, also recommended a trial on reduced dairy consumption as one of the phases of his treatment regimen. Years later, Iacono et al. (1998) performed a double-blind, cross-over study comparing cow's milk with soy milk in 65 children with chronic constipation. They reported that 44 of the 65 children had a favorable response to soy milk, while none of the children who received cow's milk had a favorable response. They concluded

> **Reduced dairy consumption can be an important component in treating encopresis**

that, in young children, chronic constipation can be a manifestation of intolerance to cow's milk.

2.3.1.4   Data Collection: Symptom Rating Sheets

Use of a structured Symptom Rating Sheet (SRS) can facilitate record keeping

The regimen required of parents and children to manage encopresis can be viewed as a complication to the already busy schedule of most families. Thus, a form for parents called the Symptom Rating Sheet (SRS), described by Christophersen (1994), can facilitate record keeping (see Appendix 2). The SRS was based upon the recommendation of Wright and Walker (1976), who had families either call the office once a week or mail in a weekly progress report. In the event that a weekly report was missed (by phone or mail) Wright and Walker called the family to check up on the child's progress. In recent years, the present authors have also asked families to e-mail weekly progress reports.

When used reliably and sent to the treatment provider's office either by e-mail with appropriate consent or brought in for each follow-up appointment, the SRS can be a quick and accurate way of assessing patient progress, making treatment plan modifications, and encouraging treatment adherence. One strategy we have used with our Symptom Rating Sheets is to instruct the parent – and the child if he/she is old enough to understand the discussion – to track the child's "Weekly Stool Volume." This refers to the child's estimated output of stool, usually using cups as a measure. By way of example, if a child has an output of about 7 cups of stool a week, for a period of at least 2–3 weeks, then a drop in estimated output to 3 cups of stool a week is a sign that the child is getting constipated again, which should alert the parent to the need for more aggressive management. "More aggressive management" means some combination of an increase in intake of dietary fiber, an increase in the child's medication, or an increase in vigorous physical exercise. Anecdotally, the best exercise appears to be swimming, although working out on a trampoline or a gymnastic/dance routine can be equally stimulating. The point is that stool output has to be maintained while the musculature in the colon heals.

As shown in Appendix 2, the symptom rating sheet asks the parent or child to record several things, including the amount and consistency of stools, bowel movements in the toilet, and daily dietary fiber intake in grams. This form can be used to watch for trends in the child's habits such as stool frequency and amount. Immediate feedback can be given on improvements as well as on warning signs that the child may be getting constipated again.

2.3.2   Methods of Treatment

2.3.2.1   Medical Treatment

The "pediatric approach" to the treatment of encopresis as originally described by Davidson (1958) and Davidson, Kugler, and Bauer (1963) included a *three-phase treatment protocol* (Christophersen & Mortweet, 2001). The first phase involved cleaning out the child's colon (catharsis) with enemas and/or giving the child large doses of mineral oil to keep the child passing stools. The second phase involved decreasing the child's dietary intake of milk and dairy products to the equivalent of one pint of whole milk a day. (Davidson had made the observation that milk, because of its low residue and high calcium content, may cause or aggravate constipation.) The objective of this phase was to reduce the need for enemas and to encourage regular bowel habits. The third phase involved continuing to encourage regular bowel movements, while gradually fading out the use of mineral oil. In 12 weeks of clinical trials with 119 severely constipated children, Davidson et al. (1963) reported a 90% success rate when using his regimen. Over the next two decades, similar procedures were employed in a number of other studies in the pediatric literature. Levine (1976) presented outcome data on 127 children with an average age of 8 years and 2 months who had primary encopresis. The children, mainly boys, were treated with a program that included counseling and education, initial bowel catharsis, a supportive maintenance program to maintain regular stooling, retraining, and careful monitoring, and follow-up. Of those children for whom 1-year outcome data were available, 51% were in remission, 27% showed marked improvement, 14% showed some improvement, and 8% were essentially unchanged. At the end of the treatment year, Levine reported that 11 difficult cases had been referred for psychiatric help. After 1 year of psychotherapy, 10 of these patients still remained in treatment. Levine's experience, and the experience of the present authors, indicates that although psychotherapy may be effective for psychological problems other than encopresis, no controlled studies have documented the effectiveness of psychotherapy as the *primary* intervention for encopresis. Rather, if a child with encopresis also presents with behavioral/emotional problems, those problems may well be amenable to psychotherapy, the same conclusion reached by van Dijk et al. (2008).

No controlled studies have documented the effectiveness of psychotherapy as a primary intervention for encopresis

In 1996, Rockney, McQuade, Days, Linn, and Alario reported long-term outcome data on 45 children treated for encopresis using a treatment regimen similar to Levine's (1976). After 4 years after treatment, 58% of the children were in remission and 29% were improved; only 13% showed no improvement. The major risk factors for treatment resistance were previous treatment for encopresis and nonretentive encopresis (i.e., no history of constipation). The longest reported follow-up on the medical management of childhood constipation is for 6.8 years (Sutphen et al., 1995). In their study, Sutphen et al. reported follow-up data on 43 children treated with an initial cleanout to remove impactions, prompted toilet sits, and laxatives (including enemas prescribed any time a child went 24 hours without a bowel movement). The majority (70%) of the children was entirely asymptomatic at follow-up, and the remaining 30% experienced intermittent mild constipation. In a study of children resistant to treatment, Landman, Levine, and Rappaport (1983) reported that continued management with a pediatric approach resulted in 57% no longer soiling at 1- to 2-year follow-ups. It appears from the treatment literature and as well as in our own clinical experience that continued reliance on a medical treatment program – in the absence of clear and contributing psychopathology – is the treatment of choice.

Major risk factors for treatment resistance include previous treatment for encopresis and nonretentive encopresis

Over the past decade, MiraLax™ (polyethylene glycol), an electrolyte-free PEG, has become a popular medication prescribed for children with chronic constipation. Bishop (2001) reported having begun prescribing MiraLax™ soon after it was marketed – initially only for patients who were noncompliant with other therapies – and then later as a first-line therapy. The most common negative side effect reported at that time was flatulence or cramping, seen in a minority of patients when fruit juices were used to mix the PEG. Later, Loening-Baucke (2002) reported on an outcome study that compared MiraLax™ with milk of magnesia (assumed *not* to be randomly assigned as there were different cell sizes in each group). At 1-, 2-, 3, and 12-month follow-ups, bowel movement frequency had increased and soiling frequency had decreased significantly in both groups. The main difference between the two groups was that none of the children refused MiraLax™, whereas 33% refused to take milk of magnesia. MiraLax™ has no taste, no loss of efficacy occurred, and does not cause clinically significant side effects. MiraLax™ has been available over the counter since 2007.

2.3.2.2 Medical-Behavioral Treatment

One of the earliest behavioral treatment programs for encopresis was offered by Wright (1975), whose treatment program consisted of initial enemas to clean the child out, followed by daily glycerin rectal suppositories if the child had not had a bowel movement that day, along with behavioral procedures designed to enhance treatment adherence, such as daily symptom and regimen recordings mailed or called into the practitioner's office on a weekly basis. Variations of this medical and behavioral treatment program have also been successful. For example, O'Brien et al. (1986) evaluated a treatment program based on the Wright (1975) program using a multiple baseline design across four children who were 4–5 years old. For two of the children, treatment with cathartics and special time with their parents (as a reinforcer for appropriate toileting) remedied their soiling accidents and increased their independent toileting in 8–11 weeks. The other two children achieved independent toileting after 32 and 39 weeks of treatment, respectively, which included positive practice, time-out, and hourly toilet sits, which had been added to the original treatment regimen.

The Stark, Owens-Stively, Spirito, Lewis, and Guevremont (1990) study furthers the research of Houts et al. (1988), who, among others, recognized the importance of the role of dietary fiber in the treatment of encopresis. Williams, Bollella, and Wynder (1995) provided a convenient summary of the recommendations of the American Academy of Pediatrics for the intake of dietary fiber. Owens-Stively (1995) also published an excellent educational guide for parents to assist them in selecting foods for their children that are high in fiber. See Appendix 1 for the fiber content of many common household foods.

2.3.2.3 Behavioral Treatment

Given the preponderance of research documenting the role that constipation plays in the etiology and management of encopresis, few authors have recommended behavioral treatment without concomitant medical treatment. A recent study examined behavioral versus medical treatment of constipation, using a prospective random assignment to alternative treatment groups (van Dijk et al., 2008). The "conventional treatment" was delivered by pediatric gastroenterologists and included a 20- to 30-minute session during which laxative treatment (PEG and, if necessary, enemas or suppositories) and a bowel diary were discussed, along with education to explain that symptoms are not harmful and common in children with functional constipation. Furthermore, children

Few authors recommend behavioral treatment without concomitant medical treatment

were instructed not to withhold stool, and motivation was enhanced by praise and small gifts from the pediatric gastroenterologists. The "behavioral treatment" was delivered by pediatric psychologists and included teaching parents behavioral procedures and doing behavioral play therapy with the child in the presence of his or her parents. The choice of behavioral play therapy was somewhat unconventional, because the published literature has seldom indicated that behavioral play therapy is an effective treatment modality for constipation. At each of their measurement intervals, there were no significant differences between the conventional and the behavioral treatments: They were equally effective.

The one other major study comparing medical treatment with behavioral treatment found somewhat similar results using prospective random assignment to three alternative treatment groups: intensive medical treatment (IMC), enhanced toilet training (ETT), and enhanced toilet training plus biofeedback (BF) (Borowitz, Cox, Sutphen, & Kovatchev, 2002). Total cure rates at the 1-year follow-up were the same for all three treatment groups, although the enhanced toilet training group had statistically significant decreases in the daily frequency of soiling for the greatest number of children.

2.3.2.4   Biofeedback Treatment

In the largest study of its kind ($n = 129$), Loening-Baucke (1995) concluded that "learning normal defecation dynamics with biofeedback training did not increase long-term recovery rates in children with chronic constipation, encopresis, and abnormal defecation dynamics above those achieved with conventional treatment alone" (p. 109). She had previously found short-term benefits of biofeedback treatment in children with constipation, encopresis, and abnormal defecation dynamics. These results are consistent with the study by Borowitz et al. (2002) comparing "intensive medical management" with "intensive medical management plus a behavior modification program," and "intensive medical management plus biofeedback training."

Biofeedback training appears not to increase long-term recovery rates

2.3.2.5   Treatment-Resistant Encopresis

The only replicated outcome data that we could identify for treatment-resistant encopresis is the protocol published by Stark et al. (1990, 1997). Stark et al. (1990) investigated behavioral group treatment for 18 children with retentive encopresis who had previously failed medical management. The small groups met over 6 sessions and focused on education about retentive encopresis and integrating behavioral parent training procedures with medical management. Parents and children were taught how to deliver an enema cleanout, how to increase the child's intake of dietary fiber, and appropriate toileting techniques. Their results indicated that children significantly increased fiber consumption by 40%, improved appropriate toileting by 116%, and decreased soiling accidents by 83% from pre- to posttreatment. Further, these treatment gains were maintained or improved on at the 6-month follow-up. Stark et al. (1997), in a study with 59 children who had failed standard medical management for retentive encopresis, implemented their treatment protocol over 6 1-hour group sessions. The treatment was essentially the same as their earlier study. For their overall sample, the number of soilings decreased 85%, the weekly frequency of parent-prompted bowel movements increased 9%, and the daily dietary fiber intake increased by 121% from pre- to posttreatment. The majority of their treatment sample (86%) had stopped soiling by the end of treatment and did not require further treatment. According to Stark et al. (1990), group interventions have several benefits: First, a group setting provides numerous parents with the same information at the same time and results in cost-effective treatment. Second, the parents who participated in the study reported feeling great relief and support in meeting other families who also had children with encopresis. In addition, the children reportedly enjoyed the group and had feelings of relief upon meeting other children with the same problem.

2.3.2.6   The Role of Psychoeducational Assessment

The vast majority of children referred for evaluation and treatment of encopresis are of normal intelligence. We found no published research indicating low IQ or learning problems in the etiology of encopresis. Rather, the available research indicates IQ and learning problems play no significant role in etiology. For example, in a recent study, 125 children presenting with constipation at a primary care setting were compared with a group of children (controls) who did not suffer from constipation. There was no difference between the two groups regarding the likelihood of having a parent or a sibling with a history of constipation or the age at which toilet training had begun. Parents of constipated children reported more difficult and painful defecation experiences than the controls, and the constipated children were more likely to express worry about future painful defecation than were the control children. The authors concluded that the various factors contributing to the etiology of constipation included genetic predisposition, premature or difficult toilet training, dietary transitions from breast milk to formula or from liquid to solid foods, painful or difficult bowel movements, beginning school, or traumatic bathroom experiences. The variables identified did not include IQ or learning problems (Borowitz et al., 2002).

Clinical experience shows no significant causal relationship between learning problems, IQ, and encopresis

This study closely corresponds with our clinical experience, which has shown no significant causal relationship between learning problems, IQ, and encopresis, and leads to our position that, in the typical child presenting with constipation and encopresis, a full battery of psychoeducational tests is neither indicated nor indeed clinically useful. If the family history and interviews with the parent(s) and the child do not suggest that low intelligence or learning issues play a significant etiological role in the child's constipation, then further assessment of these variables is likely to represent a waste of valuable resources.

2.3.3   Problems Carrying Out the Treatments

Perhaps the biggest problem in the treatment of encopresis is that children have to be motivated and encouraged to consciously think about a process – defecation – that many of their family members and friends do consciously think about.

And they have to think consciously about their diet. Children may be expected to *stop* eating certain foods (e.g., dairy products) that their family members and their friends continue to eat, and they may be expected to *start* eating foods that their family members and friends do not (have to) eat (e.g., foods high in dietary fiber).

2.3.3.1   Rewarding Children for Cooperating with the Treatment Regimen

Many practitioners instruct the parents of encopretic children to reward their children for having a bowel movement in the toilet when they should be rewarding them for cooperating with the treatment regimen. Most children with encopresis cannot just willfully have a bowel movement or they probably would not have encopresis. At the same time, it is not unusual for children to need some encouragement – and possibly rewards – in order to change or modify their diet. We prefer initially educating parents about the benefits of dietary fiber and the guideline from the American Academy of Pediatrics, that children should be eating their age plus 5 grams of fiber per day (Dwyer, 1995). We give them a handout from the Owens-Stively study (1995) explaining the benefits of dietary fiber with a listing of the fiber content of many popular foods (see Appendix 1). All we ask is that the child gets the required number of grams of fiber in their diet, preferably by eating foods they already eat and like, thus sidestepping or at least postponing the issue of getting the child to eat foods they have never eaten before.

While we do not necessarily recommend that our patients be rewarded for their intake of dietary fiber by being given fiber points as Houts et al. (1988) suggest, it is certainly a reasonable procedure. Typically, when rewarding any type of behavior, parents should use a picture menu so that their child gets to pick the reward he or she wants, when it has been earned, by pointing to the picture of the reward. One of the activities we support was actually inspired by Wright and Walker (1976), who recommended using "time with parents" as a reward. They stated that, "One of the most effective rewards, and one that is quite general in that it works with most children, is allotting them a certain period of time, say twenty or thirty minutes, at the end of the day in which their parents will do anything they ask (p. 36)." Schonwald and Sheldon (2006) made a similar statement, that "The most effective reward you can give your child is special, uninterrupted time" (p. 115).

An effective reward for children is simply spending time with their parents

2.3.4   Variations of Methods and other Stategies

2.3.4.1   The Method of Schonwald and Sheldon (2006)

Schonwald and Sheldon (2006) describe a number of steps that are very similar to those we have recommended in our clinic for years:

• **Small step stools**: Children can use a step stool to assist them in getting up on the toilet and use as leverage for their feet when they are sitting on the toilet. A narrow step stool usually will not work because children, like adults, often spread their feet apart when sitting on the toilet for better traction, which makes it easier for them to push out the bowel movement.

• **Parent modeling**: Schonwald and Sheldon (2006) call this "potty copycat," meaning children often want to do what they see their parents doing. In this case, it refers to children who insist on sitting on the "big" toilet because they see their parents doing it.

• **Involving the Preschool, Kindergarten, and School**: The most important step with schools is to ask them to refrain from giving dairy products to children who have problems with constipation. It is common for schools to request a letter from the doctor's office before limiting dairy intake. We thus

An important step with schools was asking them to refrain from giving dairy products to children who have problems with constipation

send a letter requesting that the daycare/school substitute fruit juice for dairy drinks. We also recommend parents asking the school to provide the child with more private restroom access than the public restrooms the other children use. Children in the initial stages of treatment, who are still having problems with constipation and who are still occasionally passing large stools (some of them foul smelling) are more likely to be teased by peers if they use a public restroom. If they use the restroom, say, in the nurse's office or in the faculty lounge, they are much less likely to be ridiculed by their peers.

It is important to educate preschool/ school personnel about the need for the child with encopresis to have ready access to the restroom

It is equally important to educate preschool/school personnel about the need for the child with encopresis to have ready access to the restroom. Usually schools initially will agree to this stipulation; however, when the child indicates that he/she needs to use the restroom, teachers will often ask the child to wait until break time with the rest of the class – even such a brief delay means the difference between a successful trip to the restroom and an accident.

On many occasions, we have requested the opportunity to meet with school personnel (teachers, administrators, and nurses) to educate them about encopresis, its causes, and our treatment recommendations. Just as many parents cannot understand how children can be telling the truth when they say that they do not feel a bowel movement coming, school personnel often have the same problem. In these instances, we provide a PowerPoint slide show and use Levine's (1982) demystification discussion.

A website like *Potty Training Concepts* has information and accessories for youngsters being potty trained

A website like Potty Training Concepts (http://www.pottytrainingconcepts. com) has plentiful material and accessories available for the youngster who is being potty trained. They have a "Flip Toilet Seat" that has both a regular toilet seat for teens and adults and a smaller seat for children, both of which are attached to the toilet. The child uses the small seat by simply lifting up the lid, whereas a teen or adult would lift the lid *and* the small seat to access the regular toilet seat.

2.3.4.2   Celiac Disease

With the ever-increasing popularity of gluten-free diets, parents may try exposing their children to a gluten-free diet (GFD) in the hope that it will improve their child's symptoms of constipation and encopresis. The Society of Pediatric Gastroenterology, Hepatology, and Nutrition made the very sensible recommendation: "Treatment with a GFD is recommended for all symptomatic children with intestinal histopathologic abnormalities that are characteristic of CD (Celiac Disease)" (The Constipation Guideline Committee for the North American Society for Pediatric Gastroenterology, Hepatology and Nutrition (NASPGHAN), 2006, p. 2). Based on current evidence and practical considerations, including accuracy, reliability, and cost, measurement of IgA antibody to human recombinant tissue transglutaminase (TTG) is recommended for initial testing for CD. The typical child with constipation and encopresis may have difficulty passing stools, but he or she does not have the more classic symptoms of persistent diarrhea and poor weight gain resulting from CD. There are numerous studies demonstrating that children with CD have gastrointestinal (GI) symptoms such as diarrhea with failure to thrive, abdominal pain, vomiting, constipation, and abdominal distension.

Classically, infants with celiac sprue present between the ages of 4 and 24 months with impaired growth, diarrhea, and abdominal distention. Vomiting is also common, as are pallor and edema. The onset of symptoms is gradual and follows the introduction of cereals into the diet. The velocity of weight gain slowly decreases before weight loss ensues. Some children may present with constipation, although diarrhea is more typical. Patients with severe, untreated celiac sprue may present with a short stature, pubertal delay, iron and folate deficiency with anemia, and rickets. Atypical celiac sprue is usually seen in older children or adolescents, who often have no overt features of malabsorption (Farrell & Kelly, 2002, p. 180).

In one study of undiagnosed celiac disease in children, about 1% of the 5,470 children in the study tested positive to the initial screen for celiac disease. A total of 10 children out of the 5,470 children in the study had a history of constipation and tested positive for the markers for celiac disease (Bingley et al., 2004). This would suggest that the likelihood of celiac disease being the *primary* etiological agent for constipation/encopresis in children is exceedingly low. However, since CD has only recently been included in mainstream medicine, it would not be prudent to assume that the primary-care physician had even considered celiac disease as the cause of a child's constipation/encopresis. In one of our clinical practices (over 35 years of treating literally hundreds of children with constipation/encopresis), no more than two children had documented celiac disease – and both had been previously diagnosed with the disease.

In our clinical experience few children with constipation/encopresis have celiac disease

2.3.4.3   Toilet Training School

Alison Schonwald has a "Toilet Training School" at Children's Hospital Boston which caters to youngsters who have failed at normal potty training strategies. Schonwald's Toilet Training School seems to be a major advancement in the treatment of constipation and other associated problems encountered in toilet training. The availability of seasoned professionals, intimately familiar with the strategies available for countering the problems associated with toilet training, is a refreshing addition to our armentarium for treating constipation in children. Schonwald has already treated over 450 children with toileting problems. With this kind of success, other potty training programs may well be offered by high-profile children's hospitals. This approach is distinctly different from programs offered under the sponsorship of a private individual or a local day care center. In addition, this kind of database is invaluable for collecting outcome data on the process of toilet training children.

2.4   Case Vignette: Encopresis

History: Zachary, an 8-year-old boy, was referred by his primary-care physician for treatment of constipation and encopresis. He has an enlarged colon and sometimes struggles with constipation. Reportedly, he holds his bowels. Language skills, fine and gross motor skills, and eye contact are all within normal limits. There are no sensory issues and no unusual fears. Zachary worries a lot, but there are no sleep problems. His mother reports that he can be mean and is intentionally mean to his siblings. He has friends, but at times they will not play with him. On occasion, he can be aggressive with other children.

His mother needs help in dealing with his problem – "he poops his pants." He has large caliber stools and can hold his bowel movements for a long time. Reportedly, he rarely has accidents at school because he avoids defecating until he gets home. Zachary also holds stools on alternating weekends at his dad's house until his dad sees the "expression" on his face and tells him to go poop, at which time Zachary says he will usually defecate. There are no special accommodations at school.

Assessment. The Behavior Assessment System for Children (BASC) completed by the mother had an overall clinical behavioral systems index with a T-score of 57 and a percentile rank of 78, which would be considered in the high normal range. The only clinically significant subscale for the mother was his aggression. At-Risk subscales included: conduct problems, attention problems, adaptability, social skills, and leadership. Zachary meets the DSM-IV diagnostic criteria for Encopresis in that he 1) reported passage of feces into inappropriate places (his clothing), 2) did so at least once per month for the past 3 months, 3) his chronological age is at least 4 years, and 4) the behavior is not due exclusively to the direct physiological effects of a substance (e.g., laxatives).

According to the mother's report, Zachary did not have trouble gaining weight as an infant and did not need any special vitamins or food supplements in order to gain weight. He was easy to train for urination and there is no family history of colon problems.

Case Conceptualization. This is a typical presentation for a school-age child with encopresis.

Treatment. His treatment components included:
1. Minneapolis Children's Medical Center Diet recommendations of 13 grams of dietary fiber per day, split into the three meals, and a decrease in total daily intake of milk and dairy products to no more than 12 ounces/day (Owens-Stively, 1995).
2. No need to reduce intake of natural lubricants like fried and greasy foods
3. Encourage intake of natural laxatives like pear juice and see if patient tolerates honey as a sweetener.
4. Encourage daily, vigorous exercise
5. Encourage daily intake of 6–8 glasses of nondairy liquids
6. Return to clinic in 2 weeks, then at monthly intervals.

Written treatment summaries: Levine diagram for demystification, Minneapolis Children's Medical Center Diet Handout, GI diagram, and SRS (Symptom Recording Sheets, see Appendix 2).

Outcome. At the 2-week follow-up visit, parents reported having implemented a sticker chart for rewards. Rewards included $1.00 for each day with a trip to the bathroom. At 1 month without an accident, parents promised to fix patient's GoKart. The mother had located a breakfast bar that was high in fiber which her son liked. Stool volume the first week was 1½ cups. The third week stool volume was 2¼ cups.

Recommendations were as follows: 1) add back the "green pill" (stool softener) daily; 2) split breakfast bar into halves, one half for breakfast and one half with evening meal; 3) continue to work on getting more fiber into the patient's diet. According to the SRS, the child has been averaging about 14 grams of fiber per day.

At the 6-week follow-up visit, the mother reports that Zachary is still having some accidents, but they are no longer full bowel movements. The mother is still reminding him to go to the bathroom for his bowel movements. There is less odor in his stools and more regular output.

Recommendations: (1) Reminded the mother of the need to remind the patient to use the bathroom, because he still may not be able to feel the call to stool. Asked the mother to document the time of his bowel movements because it appears that most accidents, according to mother's memory, were between 3 pm and about 6 pm. (2) Continue the green pill and prompting to use the bathroom. (3) Mentioned the option of rectal suppositories, which had been declined by both mom and patient.

At the 10-week follow-up visit, stool output per SRS was 2½ cups/week. Patient took car trip to relative several states away for Thanksgiving. The mother reported that he actually did much better over the holidays than most times in the past. They had not been as good with giving the green pill every day as they had been in the past. The mother reported that exercise is harder now with shorter days (late fall).

Recommendations: 1) Carry the high fiber bars on any long car trips and send the high fiber bars with him when he spends weekends with his dad, 2) go back to rewards for compliance with the treatment procedures (which had fallen off). The mother has a reward system, but the main components are $20 for a month without an accident and loss of $1 for each accident. Patient needs to earn more *immediate* rewards for treatment compliance.

Patient lost to follow-up, in part because of length of travel for each hospital appointment. The family lived over 100 miles away, which required an approximate 2-hour drive each way.

Note: This is a pretty typical course for an 8-year-old with encopresis living in a rural community 100 miles from the hospital. The patient made definite progress with the recommendations we made, and the family elected to discontinue their trips to the hospital. In many cases with children 8 years and older, successful treatment can take up to a year or longer. Often, once parents see that they are on the right track, they usually will not make additional appointments.

2.5   Encopresis Without Constipation

Treatment of nonretentive encopresis is not well established, making recommending an optimal course of treatment premature. Perhaps the best approach would begin with a comprehensive psychological evaluation that includes behavioral assessment techniques. Virtually all investigators who have described this subsample of children report emotional and behavioral problems and treatment resistance (e.g., Landman & Rappaport, 1985). Some of these children's soiling may be related to modifiable aspects of their social ecology. Some investigators have employed versions of the approaches outlined above and included supportive verbal therapy (Landman & Rappaport, 1985), or they have specifically taught parents how to manage their children's misbehavior

The treatment of nonretentive encopresis is not well established; thus, recommending an optimal course of treatment is premature

(Stark et al., 1990). Clearly, the various problems exhibited by this subsample (other than soiling) require some form of treatment – though the soiling itself needs direct treatment, too.

2.6   Toileting Refusal

2.6.1   Description

Children who refuse to use toilets often ask their caregiver for a diaper or a pull-up to relieve themselves in

A toileting problem that often precedes, and almost as often evolves into, functional encopresis has been variously referred to as toileting refusal or stool withholding. This typically occurs in children 3–5 years of age, so it usually would be only relevant to children in preschool and kindergarten. Often these children are not having bowel movements in their clothing, because they will ask their parent or alternative caregiver for a diaper or a pull-up and promptly relieve themselves in the garment (Christophersen & Friman, 2004).

Because the *Diagnostic and Statistical Manual* (DSM-IV; American Psychiatric Association, 1994) states that a child must be at least 48 months of age to be diagnosed with encopresis, many of these children do not, strictly speaking, have encopresis. However, there is no other DSM-IV diagnosis that adequately describes children displaying these symptoms. Toileting refusal is also not included in the DSM – Primary Care (DSM-PC), Child and Adolescent Version (American Academy of Pediatrics).

There are no known organic conditions that predispose a child to toileting refusal (Christophersen & Friman, 2004). While constipation is present in the majority of children who exhibit toileting refusal, the etiology of the constipation varies from child to child. There is also the question of whether constipation predisposes a child to toileting refusal or whether toileting refusal leads to constipation. While Borowitz et al. (2003) concluded that painful bowel movements, more than any other factor, preceded constipation, we could not locate any data that addressed the issue of which came first, the stool holding or the painful bowel movement.

2.6.1.1   Prevalence

In a prospective study of 482 children, Taubman (1997) reported that 22% experienced at least a month of stool toileting refusal. Taubman also reported that there was an association between the presence of a younger sibling and parental inability to set limits for the child and stool toileting refusal.

2.6.1.2   Etiology

Blum, Taubman, and Osborne (1997) suggested that a variety of factors could be related to toileting refusal, including early toilet training, excessive parent-child conflict, irrational fears or anxieties surrounding toileting, a difficult temperament, and hard or painful stools as a result of chronic constipation or an anal fissure. No published studies have actually examined these various factors. However, as indicated above, there are several reports that children with toileting refusal often have histories of constipation and/or painful defecation (Blum et al., 1997; Luxem et al., 1997; Taubman 1997). Toileting refusal does not appear to be caused by diagnosable behavioral conditions. In the Blum et al. (1977) study that included 54 children (27 with toileting refusal and 27 matched controls), the children with stool toileting refusal were not found to have more behavior problems than matched children who were toilet trained. This is consistent with the findings of Friman et al. (1988) for children with encopresis. One plausible possibility is learning history.

2.6.2   Diagnostic Procedures and Documentation

A psychologist whose child client has an elimination disorder should go no further with treatment until a medical evaluation has first been conducted – even children with toileting refusal. The vast majority of cases of toileting refusal may be behavioral, but there is always the possibility of some biological problem (e.g., constipation).

Psychologists working with children with an elimination disorder or toileting refusal should not proceed with treatment until a medical evaluation has been conducted

In the initial evaluation of a child with toileting refusal, the psychologist should employ a standardized behavior rating scale, completed by the parents and, if the child attends a preschool or a daycare center, by the teacher or daycare provider. If the child has problems with compliance or exhibits disruptive behaviors, address them first (or simultaneously) before addressing the toileting refusal. But, if the child has a history of constipation, there is no reason not to address the constipation (e.g., with a medication trial) in addition to any compliance issues.

A detailed toileting history is important for identifying the extent to which the child has been bothered by constipation (Christophersen & Mortweet, 2001). Because the term "constipation" has no commonly accepted definition, the clinician usually needs to ask questions about the frequency and consistency of the child's bowel movements. Simply asking if there is a history of constipation is usually not productive. The symptoms most associated with constipation include hard, pebbly stools, large stools, infrequent stools (less than one stool every 3 days), and stools that are difficult to pass. In our experience, it is not unusual for a child with toileting refusal to exhibit refusal during an office visit as well. We have witnessed attempts to hold stools during the initial office visit, including children standing with their legs twisted together, moving over to the corner of the sofa, and holding on to the arm of the sofa.

2.6.3   Treatment for Toileting Refusal

For children who are refusing to defecate in an adult toilet, Christophersen and Mortweet (2001) suggest the first step is to make certain that their stools are soft and formed. This can be accomplished by suggesting changes in diet, use of medication, or both. The dietary changes should include the addition of more dietary fiber to moisten and soften the stools and, in cases in which the child is consuming an excess of dairy products, reducing the number and amount of dairy products offered or available (Davidson, 1958). A small amount of mineral oil (1 ml per kilogram of weight) mixed with 7-Up, Sprite, or some other liquid is usually sufficient to soften stool.

For children who are refusing to defecate in an adult toilet, the first step is to ensure that their stools are soft and formed

If the child whose stools are soft and formed is still reluctant to defecate in the toilet, the child's physician can recommend the use of glycerin rectal suppositories for a period of up to 1 week. These suppositories, when given just prior to a meal (i.e., the meal closest to when the child typically has a bowel movement), help produce a bowel movement. Several bowel movements in the toilet, without discomfort, usually diminish the learned aversive properties of appropriate toileting.

By treating toileting refusal at an early age, the clinician may be able to avoid later episodes of encopresis. Many parents of children who present with encopresis report that their children had problems with constipation, toileting refusal, or both at an earlier age. It is interesting to note that the first research paper documenting normal bowel habits in children did not appear in the literature until 1984 (Weaver & Steiner). The average 1-year-old child has one or two stools per day and, by age 4, the majority of children have one stool a day, although it is not unusual for 4-year-olds to have two stools per day. Constipation should be considered if stool frequency is less than 3 times a week (Loenig-Bauke, 1996).

Luxem et al. (1997), using a combination of bowel cleanout procedure (typically enemas), high fiber foods, mineral oil therapy, and positive reinforcement for appropriate toileting, reported that the 11 children they treated were accident-free and having at least one bowel movement every 2 days during the 5 consecutive days of follow-up conducted 3–4 months after treatment. Parents reported general satisfaction with the treatment.

Schonwald and Sheldon (2006) describe a number of very similar steps to those we use with toileting refusal. We interpret toileting refusal as more of an anxiety disorder than one of noncompliance, which may well have its etiology in the constipation that probably precipitated the toileting refusal. We encourage two initial strategies.

You can desensitize a child to toilet sits by encouraging and rewarding the child for sitting on the toilet to urinate

The first strategy is to desensitize the child to toilet sits by encouraging and rewarding them (with time rewards recommended by Wright and Walker, 1976) for sitting on the toilet to urinate – both for girls and boys. We think of each of these toilet sits as another exposure with response prevention (ERP), the term used in the anxiety literature by Kendall et al. (1997) and others. Because most children urinate numerous times each day, our patients too usually relax quite readily when urinating. Other types of rewards that should be familiar to practitioners who frequently work with young children include sticker charts, dot-to-dots, grab bags, and pictures of the desired item or activity that have been cut into two or more pieces, with each piece earned by the correct behavior until the picture is complete and the reward has been earned. Some of these procedures are discussed by Schonwald and Sheldon (2006).

The second strategy is to recommend that parents allow their child to have their bowel movements in a pull-up or a diaper. The rationale for this is that we have to get the child to have regular bowel movements before commencing toilet training, in order to reduce or eliminate any chance that the child will have another painful bowel movement. Although some parents are reluctant to allow their children to have their bowel movements in a pull-up or diaper, believing it is taking a step backwards, the vast majority can be convinced to do so.

Initially, we recommend that parents reward their child for having a bowel movement in their pull-up/diaper regardless of where they are when doing so.

Then we instruct the parent(s) to reward their child only when they have a bowel movement in a pull-up/diaper when they are actually in the bathroom. Later, we instruct the parent(s) to make the rewards available only when the child defecates in the pull-up/diaper while sitting on the toilet with the lid down . And finally, we instruct parent(s) to reward only when the child defecates in the pull-up/diaper while sitting on the toilet seat with the lid up.

We also usually recommend that everything connected with toileting be kept in the bathroom that the child usually uses. That is, fresh pull-ups or diapers, diaper pail, moist towelettes, etc., should all be stored in that bathroom.

2.6.3.1 Phobia for Public Toilets

It is not uncommon for youngsters to refuse to use public toilets. The most common reason for this refusal is that children are frightened by auto-flush toilets that are loud and unpredictable. For the child with toileting refusal, we typically recommend that both the mother and the father – or any alternative caregivers – make it a point to use restrooms in public and at friends', neighbors', and relatives' houses, as well as at daycare, preschools, and schools. Often parents will themselves avoid using public restrooms as a personal preference. However, during the time that parents are dealing with a child with toileting refusal, it is best if parents openly and often use public toilets and toilets at friends, relatives, and neighbor's homes.

> **It is not uncommon for youngsters to refuse to use public toilets.**

2.6.3.2 Talking about Toileting Issues with the Child

Schonwald and Sheldon (2006) caution parents about scolding, humiliating, or punishing their children for toileting problems, and point out that constipation is rarely, if ever, a child's fault because they usually do not have control over what they eat. They also encourage parents to adopt and maintain a "no big deal" attitude about toileting accidents. We strongly encourage parents to never spend more the 5 minutes a day on *all* toilet discussions combined: Drawn-out discussions about toileting accidents rarely benefit the child who has had the accident and all too often involve letting the child know how very disappointed the adult caregivers/parents are. For large bowel accidents, we usually recommend that the parents refrain from saying anything.

> **Parents should avoid scolding, humiliating, and punishing children for toileting problems**

2.6.4 Case Vignette: Toileting Refusal

History: Jason is a 5-year-old boy whose parents asked their pediatrician for a referral because their son refused to have his bowel movements on the toilet. Assessment of Jason's accidents indicated that his mother, his maternal grandmother, and both of his sisters had had problems with constipation. The mother reported that she started toilet training Jason at about 2½ years of age, then again at 3 and at 3½ – with no luck – which was very frustrating for her. The mother reported that if she reminded Jason to use the toilet he would use it, but if left on his own, he would go ahead and have an accident. The mother had been "nagging" him about accidents (the father agrees that the mother nags) and offering small rewards for bowel movement's in the toilet. But he still wets the bed every night. The mother awakens him to change him and nag him. If he does indeed urinate in the toilet, he says that "he's a big boy." He is a good sleeper; he may ask for a drink after bedtime, but is pretty good right at bedtime. He sleeps in his own bed and is alone when he falls asleep. He likes to eat junk food like fruit rollups if he can convince his mother to purchase them.

Assessment. On the Parent BASC (Behavior Assessment System for Children) no issues were either clinically significant or at-risk. Jason displayed all of the symptoms of toileting refusal including regular stools, usually not in the toilet; preference for having his bowel movements in his underwear; over 3 years of age; and a history of constipation.

Case Conceptualization. Jason's accidents met the DSM-IV Diagnostic Criteria for Encopresis with Constipation (that was his official diagnosis). But, since he was having regular bowel movements, as opposed to a presentation of long periods of time without a bowel movement (typical for children with encopresis), he fits our definition of toileting refusal. In his official medical record, he is diagnosed with encopresis.

Treatment. Several treatment components were implemented at the first office visit including the following:

1. Make changes in the child's diet to promote soft, formed stools. This included, at a minimum, increasing his intake of dietary fiber and decreasing his intake of dairy products (including milk, cheese, cottage cheese, ice cream, custard, yogurt, and pudding) to 12 ounces/day.

2. Take all pressure off of toilet training until he has had soft, formed stools for a minimum of a 2-3 weeks or longer. A major component of toileting refusal seems to be anxiety about having another bowel movement that is painful or difficult to pass. Enough time must lapse, without any discomfort, to break any association the child may have between bowel movements and discomfort.

3. Encourage Jason to have his bowel movements in his diaper or pull-up *while* he is in the bathroom. As soon as he is finished, change and clean him up. That way, all activity related to bowel movements *occurs in the bathroom.* Every bowel movement without discomfort will help to break his association with discomfort.

4. After his stools are soft, formed, and he is having all of his bowel movements in the bathroom, begin "fading" to encourage bowel movements on the toilet. The first step is getting Jason to have his bowel movements in the pull-up or diaper while he is in the bathroom. Later, try to get him to have his bowel movements in the pull-up or diaper while sitting on the toilet.

5. Reward all cooperation with the treatment regimen – *do not hold out* and only give rewards for having a bowel movement on the toilet. Rather, give rewards for each step of the way. For example, give a reward to Jason for helping pick out good foods (high-fiber foods) in the grocery store. Since the mother reports that the patient has a bowel movement in the toilet if prompted when he shows signs of having to (holds his tummy, gets quiet, drifts away from other people), rewards are recommended following bowel movement in the toilet. If he has either a urination or a bowel accident, sterile clean up is recommended.

6. Complete the Symptom Rating Sheet (SRS) each day and bring it to each follow-up appointment.

Outcome. Jason's progress was monitored via follow-up appointments at 2 weeks, then at monthly intervals. At the first return office visit after 2 weeks,

Jason was having bowel movements in the toilet, including 3 times with no prompt from his mother. She brought in his SRS, which showed that he was averaging 8–9 grams of fiber per day and three glasses of nondairy liquid. He continued to get 2 tablespoons of MiraLax™ per day as prescribed by his primary-care physician. During the first week, Jason had 4 days with a bowel movement, and during the second week he only had 2 days without a bowel movement.

At his 6-week return appointment, on most days Jason was *not* having an accident. In the previous 4 weeks, he had had accidents only secondary to an illness. According to the SRS, he had three accidents the first week and no accidents the subsequent 3 weeks. He was averaging 9 grams of fiber per day and 3 to 3½ glasses of nondairy liquid per day. On more than half of the days in the prior 2 weeks, he had told his mother that he needed to have a bowel movement rather than needing to be "nagged."

Recommendations at that time included continuing with the 15 minutes of time with parents as a reward and fast cleanup for all bowel movements in the toilet. Recommended initiating "wipe, look, drop" to get Jason to practice wiping and to teach him how to wipe himself. Also recommended very gradual decrease in his daily dose of MiraLax™ at the rate of -10% per month and stopping the decreases if his stools got hard again or the time between stools started to increase.

2.7 Adherence and Follow-Up

2.7.1 Strategies for Maximizing Treatment Adherence

Easily understood verbal information as well as written materials should be available and given to the parent, caregiver, and child, if the child is old enough to understand. It can be as simple as putting together an encopresis packet that visually illustrates the various parts of the treatment regimen. Often, we use this packet as part of a "show-and-tell" explanation, asking families to look at and hold a suppository and enema container. Using labels that have been removed from food packaging, we demonstrate how to read them to determine fiber content. Getting patients and their caregivers comfortable with the treatment components mitigates apprehension and creates confidence, and we recommend that health-care providers spend time on this important step.

Equally as important is tailoring the regimen to the family's unique situation. Factors such as number of adults in the household, job schedules, behavioral and emotional issues, food issues, and cooperation from the school can alter the ability of the family to adhere to a particular regimen. Tailoring regimens around these issues can increase the chance of success. For example, if a child suffers from depression, those symptoms may need to be addressed first, before the child is ready to commit to either the encopresis or the toileting refusal regimen (which may require referral to another practitioner for a period of time). If a child exhibits oppositional behavioral challenges, parents may start small – choosing a few changes in the child's diet to help him or her learn to comply with requests. Or it may be as simple as beginning with basic

Easily understood verbal information as well as written materials should be available for parents, caregivers, and children

behavioral management techniques. Observing through data collection using the SRS is another way to begin with a child who exhibits resistance. The point is to design a treatment plan that has the best chance of success.

Giving the parent(s) and child the choice when to implement the various parts of treatment into their routines can improve success

Giving the parent(s) and child the ability to choose when to implement the various parts of treatment into their routines can also improve the chance of success. For example, if it is easier to incorporate taking mineral oil or MiraLax™ with an afternoon snack rather than breakfast when time is more of an issue, the treatment schedule should reflect that. Or if the time it takes to give a suppository – and wait for its effects – precludes doing it first thing in the morning, scheduling it for the evening should be considered. The timing of treatment components can be essential for encouraging compliance in older children, who are most likely embarrassed and do not want friends or others to know about their soiling problem. Discretion in giving any encopresis medications is paramount. Often the best time is when all friends or outsiders have gone home. Children will appreciate this being handled in a respectful way.

Given the family factors mentioned above, some families may not be able to handle a full treatment regimen all at once. In these cases, we recommend starting with three components first – data collection, scheduled toilet sits, and small changes in diet. The idea is to establish some immediate tangible success in these three areas. At that point, it is then easier to introduce medications such as enemas to keep the colon from becoming impacted again.

Finally, the effectiveness of reinforcing children should not be minimized. Encopresis is an embarrassing condition for children and the treatment can make it even more so. Having to have parents check and estimate the size of their stools, being asked to sit on the toilet while siblings and friends are playing, having suppositories and enemas administered, and being asked to eat food their siblings do not have to eat can be distressing to children. Therefore, any reinforcement for their cooperation for these indignities can encourage compliance to the regimen. Recommended reinforcement includes special time with a caregiver, dot-to-dots, stickers, or earning points for preferred activities or toys. Additional information about treatment adherence is provided by Christophersen and Mortweet (2001) .

2.7.2   Follow-up

Parents should know that recurrences are common, especially if the family stops the dietary recommendations or the child is ill

Parents and children need to know that encopresis treatment is a long-term project. In general, 4–6 weeks of consistent treatment may be required before any substantial improvement in encopretic symptoms is observed. Furthermore, long-term maintenance is needed to prevent recurring constipation. For these reasons, provisions need to be made for follow-up care that includes, at least during the first month of treatment, daily record keeping of the treatments and their effects. Patients may initially have to return once every 2 weeks with their Symptom Rating Sheets to discuss the successes and problems with the treatment regimen. Intermittent phone calls to answer specific questions are often helpful between appointments. Once managed, families should be made aware that recurrences are common, especially if the family stops the dietary recommendations or the child has a disruption to his or her gastric system from illness or surgery. For more complicated patients, for example, those with comorbid mental health or adherence problems, a referral to a pediatric psychologist trained in the management of encopresis is appropriate. Such psychologists are aware that encopresis stems from a medical condition, such as constipation, and are more likely to provide proper treatment focused on behavioral aspects of the problem as well as on the adherence and self-esteem issues related to embarrassment about the condition.

2.8   Summary and Conclusions

Based upon our extensive clinical experience, encopresis is probably the most frustrating presenting problem of children. Unlike almost any other conditions, families, the general public, and peers have little, if any, sympathy for the child with encopresis. And, when the child with encopresis says that they cannot feel the "call to stool" (the sense that they are about to move their bowels), almost no one believes them. Thus, most people feel that children with encopresis are soiling themselves deliberately, and that they could stop it – if they really wanted to. For many children with encopresis, this means that the next time they do feel the call to stool, they will make every attempt to prevent defecation by holding their bowels. Holding their bowels, in turn, exacerbates their condition by making them even more constipated, and the viscous cycle goes on. Early approaches, mainly the use of large quantities of mineral oil, made it harder for these children to hold their bowel movements until a more appropriate time and place, resulting in the passage of oily, orange-colored stools that most children found offensive. In the past decade or so, the availability of MiraLax™ has been a major improvement in that it is better tolerated by children for whom it is prescribed. But, at least for many of the children we have seen in our clinics, MiraLax™ alone is often not sufficient. In our recent experience, almost all of the children referred by primary-care physicians for evaluation and treatment of encopresis were already taking MiraLax™ and were still having problems with fecal soiling.

While MiraLax™ can easily be prescribed within the time constraints of a primary care practice (and is now available over the counter), the rest of the available treatment protocols cannot. Encopresis is a very heterogeneous ailment: Some children with encopresis respond to a brief trial on MiraLax™, get their stooling habits established, and have no further problems. However, the children referred to pediatric psychologists are often more complicated cases and require different regimens depending on how they present. Perhaps the most difficult aspect of treating constipation for the child with encopresis is that, when they are chronically constipated, they often do not have much of an appetite, so any attempt to make changes in their diet to include more dietary fiber and fewer dairy products is often met with real resistance on the part of the child. But, without increases in dietary fiber, many of these children do not improve. So, the pediatric psychologist may need to devise strategies, in cooperation with the parent(s), to encourage the child to try out new foods. The strategy we have adopted is to focus, at least in the first months of treatment, on getting the child to eat high-fiber foods that they like and have eaten before. As their constipation improves and their appetite improves, it becomes less of

Encopresis is one of the most frustrating presenting problems of children

Referrals for toileting refusal have increased significantly over the past two decades, while referrals for encopresis have been decreasing

a struggle to get them to try new foods.

Over the past decade or two, referrals for toileting refusal have increased significantly, while referrals for encopresis have been decreasing. That may well be due to the fact that the pediatric psychologist has a lot more to offer in the treatment of toileting refusal (at least in part because the treatment includes many components not typically offered through a traditional GI service). And, conversely, a hospital-based GI service may be a much more appropriate venue for treatment of encopresis in the older child (8 years and older), who has a much longer history of problems with constipation and whose medication needs to be a more integral part of the treatment.

Finally, going over the causes and treatments for encopresis takes time, something most primary-care physicians do not have. Some GI clinics have now established teams composed of GI doctors and GI nurse practitioners. And, in a limited number of settings, the team may even have an experienced pediatric psychologist. Even going over Levine's (1982) demystification diagram takes time, and going over the dietary changes necessary to maintain adequate colonic functioning takes even more time. In this respect, the pediatric psychologist is well suited to diagnose, evaluate, and manage constipation and encopresis if they have had adequate supervised clinical training. Thanks in large part to the efforts of Wright (1975) and of Wright and Walker (1976), the management of encopresis is one of the first demonstrations of evidence-based treatments. In McGrath et al.'s (2000) review, there is enough efficacious literature to merit implementation of treatment protocols at their current level. And, there is certainly much that needs to be studied about encopresis.

Nocturnal Enuresis

3.1 Description

3.1.1 Terminology and Definition

Experts have supplied multiple definitions of enuresis during its history as an affliction of childhood. The term itself, derived from the Greek word *ourein*, which means to urinate, was first used during the 19th century. For much of the 20th century, experts defined enuresis as the repeated and involuntary release of urine into or onto a location not suited for that purpose in children older than 3 years. This age limit corresponded with the age at which most children were believed to be continent at night (Powell, 1951; Schaefer, 1995). Research on the attainment of continence, however, revealed that this level was set too low (e.g., Berk & Friman, 1990), and the American Psychiatric Association (APA) revised the age limit upwards to 5 years. It also distinguished between primary cases, in which the child has never attained continence, and secondary cases, in which the child attains but fails to sustain continence.

The diagnostic criteria for enuresis as described in the Diagnostic and Statistical Manual for Mental Disorders, Fourth Edition (DSM-IV; American Psychiatric Association, 1994) may be found in Table 4.

Table 4
DSM-IV Criteria for 307.6 Enuresis

Enuresis

A. Repeated voiding of urine into bed or clothes (whether voluntary or intentional).

B. The behavior is clinically significant as manifested by either a frequency of twice a week for at least 3 consecutive months or the presence of clinically significant stress or impairment in a social, academic (occupational) or other important area of functioning.

C. Chronological age is at least 5 years (or equivalent developmental level).

D. The behavior is not due exclusively to the direct physiological effects of a substance (e.g., laxatives) or a general medical condition except through a mechanism involving constipation.

Specify type
    Nocturnal Only
    Diurnal Only
    Nocturnal and Diurnal

Reprinted with permission from the *Diagnostic and statistical manual of mental disorders, Fourth Edition* (© 1994) American Psychiatric Association.

3.1.2   Epidemiology

As many as 25% of boys and 15% of girls were enuretic at age 6, and as many as 8% of boys and 4% of girls at age 12

Estimates of the prevalence of enuresis vary widely, partly because of the samples used to generate the estimates, and partly because of changing definitions. For example, if the definition extends down to age 3, then estimates of prevalence will be far larger than if it extends only to age 5. Nonetheless, even the most conservative research-based estimates show enuresis to be a very common problem among children. For example, the National Health Examination Survey reported as many as 25% of boys and 15% of girls were enuretic at age 6, with as many as 8% of boys and 4% of girls still enuretic at age 12 (Gross & Dornbusch, 1983; see also Foxman, Valdez, & Brook, 1986). Prevalence studies from outside the United States estimate that at least 7% of all 8-year-old children wet their beds with an approximate two-to-one ratio of boys over girls (Verhulst et al., 1985). Estimates of the percentage of cases that are primary according to the definition given above range from 80% to 90% (e.g., Mellon & Houts, 1995).

3.1.3   Course and Prognosis

Enuresis is a relatively benign condition that resolves in virtually every case, even without treatment

Although enuresis can impose social and psychological burdens on afflicted children and their families, it is, in itself, a relatively benign condition and one that resolves over time in virtually every case, even without treatment. A 15% spontaneous cure rate is well documented (Forsythe & Redmond, 1974). The most problematic potential physiopathological outcome is urinary tract infection, a rare correlate, and one that is more likely due to improper hygiene in response to incontinence than to the incontinence itself. Of much greater concern are the psychological outcomes that can result from how the enuretic child is treated by important others, most notably by family members, teachers, and peers. Enuresis in the high school years and adulthood exists, but rarely, with the exception of increased incidence at the onset of the geriatric years. Unfortunately, enuretic children who do not receive effective treatment cannot volitionally stop or reduce their accidents: The problem is beyond their control. If the social response to their accidents is punishing in any way, then the children are in effect being punished for a behavior they cannot control.

The psychological sequalae resulting from the way parents, siblings, teachers, and others respond to enuresis are far more consequential than the enuresis itself

One subtle form of punishment is treating enuretic children as if they are qualitatively somehow different from nonenuretic children

Examples of punishment from parents include reduced privileges, fluid restriction, criticism, corporal punishment, and the promise of unattainable rewards (e.g., the child is promised a bicycle if bedwetting stops). Peers engage in ridicule, rumoring, and ostracism, while teachers often respond to enuresis with criticism, reduced privileges, and drawing social attention to the condition. An example of a more pervasive and more subtle form of punishment is the tendency to treat enuretic children as if they are qualitatively somehow different from nonenuretic children. Thus, although enuresis almost always resolves without treatment, untreated cases can last for 10 or more years. And if, during those years, afflicted children are exposed to direct or indirect punishment, their psychological prognosis could be adversely affected.

Most empirical research shows that enuretic children as a group exhibit a slight elevation in other psychological problems, but that only a small minority thereof are significantly impaired (e.g., Friman, Handwerk, Swearer,

McGinnis, & Warzak, 1998; Shaffer, Gardner, & Hedge, 1984). Therefore, from the currently reigning biobehavioral perspective on enuresis, the prognosis for enuretic children appears to be quite good with two caveats: (1) all forms of punishment should be prevented or eliminated, and (2) timely and effective treatment must be made available (Friman, 2008).

Improvement is reflected in gradual reductions in the volume and frequency of accidents. Severe cases can involve multiple high-volume accidents at night, whereas cases nearing resolution may involve only one or two accidents a month. A few studies suggest that the volume of urine, as indexed by the size of the urine stain, is a more sensitive measure of progress (or lack thereof) toward continence than wet or dry nights as such (Ruckstuhl, 2003). Although children with severe cases can take longer to achieve full continence, no evidence indicates that their prognosis is in any other way problematic.

3.1.4   Differential Diagnosis

The differential diagnosis for enuresis includes multiple true physiopathological conditions that, although not prevalent, may cause urinary incontinence in children (e.g., Cohen, 1987; Gross & Dornbusch, 1983). A representative list includes the following:

- Urinary obstructions (e.g., bladder stones, pelvic tumors)
- Urinary tract infection (more often in girls)
- Extreme constipation, megacolon
- Diabetes
- Seizure disorders
- Lower urinary tract obstruction
- Neurogenic bladder resulting from myelodysplasia, trauma, or other neurological disorders
- Physiological genitourinary abnormalities
- Congenital malformation of the urinary tract
- Sleep apnea

The differential diagnosis for enuresis includes multiple true physiopathological conditions that, although not prevalent, may cause primary incontinence in children

Although all of these medical causes of enuresis have the potential to cause or be complicated by psychological problems, none is a primary psychological concern, nor is any one thereof the primary object of psychological assessment instruments. Additionally, all medical causes of enuresis have a higher probability of leading to serious medical sequelae, if left untreated, than enuresis itself does. For these reasons, and for those reasons described in the assessment section below, we recommend that all enuretic children be evaluated medically before psychological treatment is begun in earnest. Furthermore, although the medical causes include multiple medical specialty concerns, the initial appointment should be with a primary care practitioner who is better trained than a psychologist to determine whether medical specialties may be needed.

3.1.5   Comorbidities

ADHD is the only distinct psychological condition for which persuasive empirical support is available for a comorbid relationship with enuresis.

Enuretic children as a group have more psychological problems than children in general; however, this higher rate of problems is not considered clinically significant and it tends to diminish following successful treatment

Although enuretic children as a group exhibit a slightly elevated level of psychological problems in general, the elevation is not considered clinically significant, and it tends to diminish following successful treatment (Friman et al., 1998; Moffatt, 1989; Shaffer et al., 1984). Recent studies regarding ADHD, however, have demonstrated a significant relationship between ADHD and enuresis (e.g., Baeyens et al., 2004; Shreeram, He, Kalaydijian, Brothers, & Merikangas, 2009). These studies suggest that the co-occurrence of the two conditions is approximately 30% greater than chance expectations. This comorbid relationship is interesting from a theoretical and clinical perspective because the modest elevations in other psychological problems have routinely been described as resulting from the enuresis itself (Friman et al., 1998; Moffatt, 1989; Shaffer et al., 1984). And as indicated above, they tend to recede as the enuresis itself diminishes. Obviously this would not be the case with ADHD, a condition that has an independent etiology and would likely persist after the enuresis had been remedied (Barkley, 1997). Additionally, the constellation of problems associated with ADHD could interfere with treatment regimens for enuresis.

3.1.6   Diagnostic Procedures and Documentation

The most important aspect of the diagnostic process for enuresis is to determine the timing and frequency of urinary accidents. One obvious reason for this is the temporal distinction between *nocturnal* and *diurnal* enuresis. One not-so-obvious reason is that, as children with nocturnal enuresis attain continence, their accidents tend to occur nearer their wakeup times, that is, they learn to inhibit urination for increasingly longer periods of time during the night. Timing is also important in children with diurnal enuresis because the typical times at which accidents occur can be used to establish times for scheduled bathroom visits.

Recent research has focused on the size of the nightly urine stain as a variable that can contribute to the assessment process

An obvious reason for considering the frequency of accidents is that it involves an aspect of the primary diagnostic criteria. To meet criteria, accidents must occur at least twice a week for at least 3 consecutive months. A not-so-obvious reason is that frequency of accidents is correlated with functional bladder capacity (FBC), a core component of the biobehavioral model of enuresis (e.g., Muellner, 1961; Starfield, 1967; Troup & Hodgson, 1971). For example, multiple nightly accidents would suggest significantly reduced FBC, whereas accidents occurring only a few times throughout the week would suggest higher capacity. Recent research also introduced the size of the nightly urine stain as a variable that definitely contributes to the assessment process (e.g., Ruckstuhl, 2003). Specifically, it can be an indicator of an incontinent child's proximity to continence: The smaller the spot, the closer the proximity. It can also be used to gauge treatment progress.

There are multiple other aspects of the diagnostic process, perhaps the most important of which is the medical examination (discussed in the section on differential diagnosis) which all enuretic children should have before biobehavioral treatment is begun in earnest. The examination should include a urinalysis (UA). The medical examination is necessary to screen for the physiopathological variables and for conditions associated with enuresis, which, as describedabove, are rare but very real and must be ruled out medically before any primary treatment plan is implemented (Christophersen & Friman, 2004; Friman, 2008; Gross & Dornbusch, 1983; Mellon & Houts, 1995).

This emphasis on the medical examination should be construed as enhancing rather than undermining the role of the psychologist. As discussed later, the theoretical model of enuresis with the most empirical support (by a very wide margin) is the *biobehavioral* one. This model unites biological, behavioral, and psychological perspectives into a unified view of the child – one that sets the stage for a synergistic partnership between psychologist and physician. It is our experience that physicians prefer to work with psychologists who respect the medical dimensions of presenting problems and are more likely to consult with and refer to those that do (Christophersen, 1982a,b).

Although medical involvement takes place early in the sequence of events in the diagnostic process, there are some psychological aspects that can be pursued immediately. For example, the parents and the child probably have dealt unsuccessfully with enuresis for an extended period and may thus have become pessimistic about the potential for progress. Also, because a residue of characterological and psychopathological interpretations (see discussion below) of enuresis remain in Western cultures, it is possible the parents and the child have misinterpreted the problem. Therefore, the diagnostic process should include some potentially therapeutically reactive features, such as optimism about outcome and deconstruction of antiquated notions that sometimes lead to blaming or shaming the child (or the parent!).

Both parents and children frequently misinterpret the meaning and significance of enuresis

The process should include questions derived from the above section on the definition (e.g., primary vs. secondary) as well as possible etiological factors derived from the biobehavioral section below (e.g., family history). Some screening for mental health problems should also be included (e.g., behavior checklists, related inquiry). As discussed previously, comorbid mental health problems are much more likely to be caused by the personal, familial, and social *responses* to enuresis than they are to be a cause thereof. Nonetheless, if the child presents with mental health problems, these should be addressed in the ultimate treatment plan.

In addition to addressing potential medical and psychological complications of enuresis, the diagnostic process should also address three other very important topics. First, all sources of punishment for wetting should be identified and proscribed. A direct way is simply to admonish parents not to punish their children and an indirect way is to show them that wetting accidents lie beyond their child's immediate control. Second, the motivation, abilities, and resources of the parents should be determined. If parents are minimally motivated and/or have limited abilities or resources (e.g., single working parent, handicapped parent), the number of treatment components they will be able to implement may be limited. Third, the child's motivation should be assessed. Optimal treatment plans involve multiple components and require compliance from the child for completion of most steps. An unmotivated or noncompliant child is difficult to treat with any method known to cure enuresis. Fortunately, the nature of enuresis itself usually contributes to the afflicted child's motivation: With the increase in the number of missed pleasant experiences (e.g., overnight stays at friends, camp) and unpleasant experiences encountered (e.g., wetness, social detection, embarrassment), motivation naturally increases as well.

Psychologists can significantly help children by immediately identifying and then proscribing all types of punishment applied in earlier attempts to eliminate the problem

3.2   Theories and Models of Enuresis

3.2.1   Historical

A review of the history of enuresis shows that the Egyptians were the first to document it as a medical disorder as early as 1550 BC. Thomas Phaer, the author of the first book on pediatrics written in the English language, described it as a disease of the "humors" and the bladder (Glicklich, 1951). The early theories of enuresis yielded treatments whose harshness appear to have been limited only by the creativity of the ancient therapists and their tolerance for inflicting unpleasantness on young children in order to secure the desired outcome. Here is a plausible scenario: A 10-year-old boy wakes on a cold morning in a fragrant, urine-soaked bed, having slept on sheets that cannot be laundered readily or properly because washing machines and household electricity have yet to be invented. All washing is done by hand, when it is done at all. He realizes that once again he has wet his bed, even though he fervently prayed before going to bed that he would not. Upon his parent's discovering his accident, they verbally and physically punish him. Later that day, they take him to a village physician who describes the boy's condition as one involving a disease resulting from defective moral and character development. The physician then prescribes a treatment, selected from a range of harsh options, including cauterizing and/or binding the penis, burning the sacrum, burning the buttocks or forcing the ingestion of the minced testicles of a rodent (Glicklich, 1951). The physician also recommends that the boy's parents continue to punish accidents, and that they use a shaming procedure such as forcing the boy to wear his urine-soaked pajamas for the entire day or hanging his urine-stained bedclothes from the window for all passersby to see.

A review of ancient approaches to enuresis indicates that this experience would not be an unusual one for a bedwetting boy of that day (Glicklich, 1951). The life of a child with a bedwetting problem would have been pretty bleak indeed. In fairness to the parents and to ancient therapists, however, the health-based consequences of prolonged bedwetting could be severe, due to difficulties posed by cleaning urine-stained bedding and clothes, the limited capacity to manage hygiene, and the very limited capacity to control infections of all types. Additionally, parents and therapists were guided by a societal interpretation of urinary incontinence which almost certainly made harsh treatment seem appropriate.

Urinary continence is a foundational component of civilization and socialization across almost all cultures. Failure to attain it after a certain age is viewed as a defect, with the severity of interpretations ranging from psychopathology to flawed moral and character development. That such stigmatizing interpretations are still operative, even with abundant research showing that urinary incontinence rarely involves pathology of any kind – not to mention flaws in morality or character – suggests that the incontinent child of yesteryear was probably routinely seen as guilty of a serious breach of conduct by the court of family and public opinion.

3.2.2 Psychopathological

The onset of the 20th century inaugurated an evolution in treatment for enuresis. For the most part, professionals began to abandon earlier harsh treatments in favor of modern approaches that were more humane from a physical perspective, though they remained problematic from a psychological vantage point. For example, with the rise of Freudian psychodynamics came psychopathological characterizations of common childhood problems such as enuresis (e.g., Sperling, 1994). Although no actual science was ever presented to support this position, it has not yet become entirely extinct. Even late into the 20th century, dynamically oriented clinical literature still characterized enuresis as a symptom of some underlying, unresolved psychosexual conflict and recommended treatments that targeted the conflict with verbal methods, rather than targeting the urinary accidents with skills training (e.g., Sperling, 1994). Some of this literature took the extreme position that, even after enuretic children had become fully continent, they were still somehow inherently enuretic (Browne, 1986). In other words, enuresis was interpreted as a psychopathological condition, and urinary accidents were seen as mere symptoms of a much larger underlying problem not defined by these accidents. Such positions place a heavy interpretative burden on afflicted children. Even after shedding themselves of their wetting problem, they were still at risk for being the object of a debilitating interpretation, one suggesting that the appearance of normality evoked by the elimination of accidents is illusory, and that the specter of pathology, although subtle, is still a significant part of their psychological makeup. It is difficult to fathom how afflicted children could extricate themselves on their own from this imbroglio of pathological interpretation. However, the almost (but not quite) complete substitution of the biobehavioral for the psychopathological model has made life substantially easier for enuretic children across the industrialized world.

3.2.3 Biobehavioral

Although the information given above paints a pessimistic picture for the enuretic child, professionals, parents, and the public have gradually abandoned their pathological, characterological, and moral views of child urinary incontinence and adopted more benign interpretations derived from a biobehavioral model (Christophersen & Friman, 2004; Friman, 2008; Houts, 1991). This shift in perspective was brought about by a confluence of biobehavioral research programs that emphasized the physiology of urination, genetics, maturational delay, anitdiuretic hormones, sleep dynamics, learning and modeling, and life events rather than psychopathology, morality, and character. Each of these dimensions of the biobehavioral model are discussed in the respective sections that follow.

3.2.3.1 Physiology of Urination

Some knowledge of the physiology of urination is necessary to understand the mechanics of urinary incontinence and the logic behind the empirically supported treatments of it. A complex physiological system governs urination, its

Table 5
Four Physiologic Steps to Urinary Control

1. Child detects contractions of the bladder resulting from filling
2. Child contracts pelvic floor muscles to elevate the bladder neck
3. Child maintains contraction of the pelvic floor muscles until he or she is in a location appropriate for urination
4. Once in an appropriate location, the child relaxes pelvic floor muscles thus allowing urination to proceed

Some knowledge of the physiology of urination is necessary to understanding the mechanics of urinary incontinence

central component being the bladder. The bladder is an elastic hollow organ resembling an upside down water balloon with a long narrow neck; it has two primary mechanical functions: the storage and release of urine (Vincent, 1974). Extended storage and timed, intentional release into an appropriate receptacle are the defining properties of urinary continence. Contraction of the bladder walls and relaxation of the bladder neck precede elimination, but the body of the bladder is composed of smooth muscle, and its nerve supply is autonomic. Therefore, the bladder cannot be controlled directly; one cannot "will" the bladder walls to contract or the neck to relax. The autonomic basis of bladder contraction and relaxation presents an apparent paradox, because the essence of complete continence is the exercise of personal control over bladder functions.

The paradox is resolved by other components of the urogenital system that in fact can be directly controlled so that a child can learn to time and locate urination appropriately. These components include three large muscle groups, sometimes referred to as pelvic floor muscles, including the thoracic diaphragm, lower abdominal musculature, and pubococcygeus (anterior end of the levator ani) (Muellner, 1960, 1961). Deliberate urination at all levels of bladder filling involves a coordination of these three muscle groups resulting in intraabdominal pressure being directed to the bladder neck. This coordinated action relaxes and lowers the bladder neck, resulting in reflexive contractions of the bladder body, opening of its internal and external sphincters, and finally bladder emptying.

Urine retention generally involves a retrograded version of this process. That is, except during imminent or actual urination, the pelvic floor muscles remain in a state of static partial contraction or tonus, which maintains the bladder neck in an elevated position and keeps the sphincter muscles closed (Vincent, 1974). Even after urination has begun, contraction of the pelvic floor muscles can abruptly raise the bladder neck and interrupt urine flow, though this requires some training and concentrated effort. The capacity to terminate and reinitiate urination is a prerequisite for Kegel exercises, a treatment method discussed later in the book (Kegel, 1951).

3.2.3.2 Genetics

Of all the research on the causes of enuresis, studies devoted to family history and genetics have likely done more to persuade parents and professionals that urinary incontinence in children is not a moral, characterological, or psychopathological concern. The knowledge that enuresis is generally an inherited condition makes it much more difficult for parents to justify any of their own disparaging interpretations of their child's incontinence, to accept such interpretations from others, or to use them as a rationale for punishing urinary accidents. As an inherited condition, enuresis seems much more likely to set the stage for sympathy than enmity.

Research on the genetics of enuresis is confined primarily to the nocturnal variety, and it reveals that the probability of enuresis increases as a function of closeness or number of blood relations with a positive history (e.g., Bakwin, 1973; Kaffman & Elizur, 1977). These early findings suggested a genetic connection, though some theorists, seemingly wed to a psychological perspective, argued against genetic transmission, asserting instead that families transmitted tolerant *attitudes* toward bedwetting, not actual enuretic "genes" (e.g., Kanner, 1972). No empirical evidence was supplied to buttress this claim, however. Quite the contrary, the related research showed that, even in settings where family customs played a minimal role in child development, such as in the Israeli kibbutzim, there was a high correlation between family history and enuresis (Kaffman & Elizur, 1977). More recent research on the the actual genetics of enuresis has identified some likely chromosomes as well as modes of transmission (Arnell et al., 1997).

Studies devoted to family history and genetics have helped dissuade both parents and professionals that urinary incontinence in children is not a moral, characterological, or psychological problem

3.2.3.3 Maturational Delay

The general heritability of enuresis raises the question of what exactly is inherited. One line of research on the developmental status and trajectory of enuretic children suggests maturational delay with multiple manifestations. For example, enuretic children exhibit reduced FBC, that is, the frequency and volume of their urination resembles that of much younger children (Scharf & Jennings, 1988). As another example, children with lower developmental levels at the ages of 1 and 3 years are significantly more likely to develop enuresis than children with higher developmental levels (Fergusson, Horwood, & Shannon, 1986). Also, there is an inverse relationship between birth weight and enuresis at any age, and enuretic children tend to lag slightly behind their nonenuretic peers in Tanner sexual maturation scores, bone growth, and height (Gross & Dornbusch, 1983). The increased prevalence of enuresis in boys also suggests maturation lag because boys generally have a slower rate of development than girls throughout childhood and adolescence (Fergusson et al., 1986; Gross & Dornbusch, 1983; Verhulst et al., 1985). The differential occurrence of enuresis between boys and girls is so robust that one group of investigators has recommended elevating the age cutoff of diagnosis for boys to 8 years, while continuing with the age of 5 years for girls (Verhulst et al., 1985). Finally, there is the 15% annual spontaneous remission rate consistent with the notion that enuretic children lag behind in the acquisition of continence, a developmental milestone for all children (Forsythe & Redmond, 1974). Despite the apparent maturational lag in many – perhaps most – enuretic children, their scores on standardized intellectual tests usually lie within the average range (Gross & Dornbusch, 1983). Thus, the maturational lag appears more anatomical and/or physiological than intellectual, and its cardinal expression is delayed bladder control.

3.2.3.4 Functional Bladder Capacity (FBC)

As indicated above, a core component of the maturational delay associated with enuresis is diminished FBC (Scharf & Jennings, 1988). FBC refers to the volume of urine released during the act of urination, and research distinguishes it from true bladder capacity (TBC), which depends on the structure of the bladder and the volume of urine it can actually hold (Troup & Hodgson, 1971). FBC is established in various ways, including the higher volume in either of the first two voidings after ingestion of a specified water load (e.g., 30 ml/kg body weight), the average of all voidings in 24 hours, or the average of all voidings in 1 week. Multiple studies have shown that the FBC of enuretic children is diminished compared with their nonenuretic siblings and peers (Muellner, 1961; Starfield, 1967; Troup & Hodgson, 1971), though no studies have shown a significant difference involving TBC (Troup & Hodgson, 1971). Generally, research on FBC suggests enuretic children are likely to urinate more frequently with less volume than their nonenuretic peers and siblings. In this respect, the urinary pattern of enuretic children has been compared to that of very young children – which supports the case for maturational delay. .

3.2.3.5 Antidiuretic Hormone (ADH)

Research on ADH (arginine vasopression) offers another potential biobehavioral etiological variable, although one not necessarily associated with maturational delay. That research suggests that enuretic children may not produce sufficient amounts of it to control urination during sleep. ADH causes the kidneys to increase the concentration of urine by increasing reabsorption of free water in the renal-collecting duct. Theoretically, serum ADH levels increase at night and thereby protect sleep from urinary urgency and facilitate nocturnal continence. One line of research has shown that a subset of enuretic children fail to exhibit the normal rhythm of ADH secretion and perhaps wet their beds as a result of increased urine production during sleep (e.g., Norgaard, Pedersen, & Djurhuss, 1985).

Another line of research provides indirect support for the role of reduced ADH in enuresis by showing that desmopressin (DDAVP), an analogue of ADH, can reduce urinary accidents in enuretic children (e.g., Dimson, 1986; also see DDAVP under the Treatment section below). Whether the effectiveness of DDAVP lies in the restoration of insufficient nocturnal ADH or is merely the result of decreased urine volume (due to increased concentration) is presently unknown (Houts, 1991; Key, Bloom, & Sanvordenker, 1992).

3.2.3.6 Sleep Dynamics

The medical literature classifies nocturnal enuresis (there is no relationship between sleep and diurnal enuresis) as a parasomnia and therefore, by definition, a sleep problem. But whether it occurs as a function of problematic sleep has yet to be established. Unfortunately, the terms for the two primary sleep variables of scientific interest, *arousability* and *deep sleep*, are understood and used differently by sleep researchers and parents. For the researcher, depth of sleep is measured by noting changes in electroencephalogram (EEG) readings, and arousability is determined by the amount of sleep-disturbing stimuli (e.g., noise, physical touch) required to awaken a child. For parents, most of whom have little technical knowledge of EEG readings and stages of sleep, depth of sleep corresponds to the researcher version of arousability. A reflection of the problem resulting from the differential use of these terms is that most parents of enuretic children regard enuresis as an outcome of overly deep sleep (Friman, 2008). An influential body of research, however, shows that wetting episodes occur in all stages of nonrapid eye movement (NREM) sleep. The probability of their occurrence appears to be a function of the amount of time spent in each stage, and enuretic children do not appear to spend an abnormal amount of time in any stage of sleep (Mikkelson & Rapoport, 1980). Thus depth of sleep, as determined by EEG readings, does not appear to be a significant factor. Enuretic episodes also rarely occur during REM sleep, so that thematically related dreams, such as dreaming of urinating, may be a result rather than a cause of wetting.

Recent research suggests enuretic children are more difficult to awaken than their nonenuretic peers

Arousability, however, also may be a contributing factor. The central question surrounding arousability is whether enuretic children are more difficult to awaken than their nonenuretic peers. Although early research was inconclusive, more recent research persuasively suggests that this is indeed the case (Gellis, 1994).

3.2.3.7   Learning and Modeling

Research has supplied no direct evidence that learning plays a significant role in the development of enuresis, although it does in the treatment of enuresis. Almost all nocturnal enuretic events occur while the children are asleep, so that the probability of *volitional* urination is limited. Additionally, the large number of cases that are primary (no previous continence) also weighs against the role of learning in the development of enuresis.

3.2.3.8   Stressful Life Events

As indicated in the section on definition, enuresis is subdivided into primary and secondary types; with the secondary type occurring after a period of continence has been established. 10% to 20% of all cases involve the secondary type, and these are often attributed to stressful life events that cause some regression or loss of continence skills (Fritz & Anders, 1979; Gross & Dornbusch, 1983). One life event that can cause enuresis is the onset of a psychotropic medication regimen (Jose, 1981). Other life events that have been said to cause secondary enuresis include any cause of significant distress for children, such as hospitalization, parental divorce, moving to a new home, and the birth of a sibling. In one study, such events occurred in the month before the onset of secondary enuresis in 81% of cases (Fritz & Anders, 1979). Despite these suggestive data, and the frequent attempts to link psychosocial variables to the precipitation of enuresis, the majority opinion is that the etiology of enuresis is primarily biological (e.g., Christophersen & Friman, 2004; Fergusson et al., 1986; Friman, 2008).

3.3   Treatment for Enuresis

3.3.1   Methods of Treatment

As we have seen above, therapists of antiquity often used harsh methods in their attempts to treat enuresis. Unfortunately for enuretic children, although therapists ultimately cam to abandon such harsh physical methods, they did so only gradually. Parents often bypassed therapists and devised physical treatments on their own. So throughout the 20th century, enuretic children were still subjected to a wide variety of folk treatment methods that, while not meeting the degree of harshness of those prescribed by therapists of antiquity, could often be physically unpleasant and wholly unnecessary. For example, beds were raised, sleeping positions were altered, garments were changed, and potions were ingested (Schaefer, 1995). Such methods are scarce now, but one aversive method has survived and still flourishes: Professionals often prescribe, and parents even more often practice, fluid restriction at bedtime for enuretic children. In fact, fluid restriction may be the most widely used method for treatment of enuresis. Yet no scientific study has ever linked fluid ingestion to diurnal or nocturnal accidents (unless the ingestion was irresponsibly large).

No scientific study has ever linked fluid ingestion to diurnal or nocturnal accidents

Once harsh physical treatments from antiquity had been abandoned, psychotherapy, derived from the psychopathology model described above, became a dominant form of treatment. As the biobehavioral model emerged, however, investigators derived conditioning-type treatments from it, and because these treatments rapidly produced large results (e.g., Mowrer & Mowrer, 1938) – while psychotherapy slowly produced small results, when it produced any results at all (e.g., DeLeon, & Mandell, 1966) – treatment providers all but abandoned psychotherapy as a treatment modality for enuresis. The success of the biobehavioral model produced a veritable paradigm shift in the treatment of enuresis. A minor attempt to use cognitive therapy to treat enuresis has been reported (Ronen, Wozner, & Rahav, 1992), but the results were questionable (Houts, 2000).

Controlled evaluations of the urine alarm indicates this relatively simple device to be 65% to 80% effective

The chief conditioning type treatment for enuresis involves the so-called urine alarm and if not the first, then certainly the foremost, early user thereof was Herbert Mowrer (Mowrer & Mowrer, 1938). Since the mid 1970s, psychological research on enuresis in children has been dominated by evaluations of urine alarm treatment and other biobehavioral methods, which have been used independently (Friman, 2008), but are mostly used to supplement the alarm (Houts, 2000; Mellon & McGrath, 2000). Controlled evaluations of the urine alarm indicate that this relatively simple device is 65–80% effective, with a duration of treatment around 5–12 weeks, and a 6-month relapse rate of 15–30% (Friman, 2008; Mellon & McGrath, 2000). Most of this research has been conducted using the bed device and, less frequently, the pajama device. Treatment involving the alarm used alone, or in strategic combinations with other treatment components, has been established as effective according to the rigorous criteria established by the Clinical Psychology Division of the American Psychological Association (Mellon & McGrath, 2000). The sections below describe alarm-based treatments in terms of method, mechanism, and outcome; we then describe the supplemental components with the most empirical support because they have been shown to be effective when used either in isolation or as part of a treatment package.

3.3.1.1   Bed Devices

The urine alarm uses a moisture-sensitive switching system that, when closed by contact with urine seeped into pajamas or bedding, completes a small voltage electrical circuit and activates a stimulus that is theoretically strong enough to cause waking (e.g., buzzer, bell, light, or vibrator). Early bed devices used two aluminum foil pads, the top one of which was perforated, with a cloth pad between them. More current devices use a rubberized pad. When a sufficient amount of urine penetrates the pad to activate the sensor, the alarm sounds. In principle, the awakened child turns off the alarm and manages their accident independently or by summoning parents for assistance. In practice, the alarm often alerts parents first, who manage the accident jointly with the child by wakening and then guiding him or her through the training steps (Friman, 2008).

3.3.1.2 Pajama Devices

Pajama devices are similar in function, yet simpler in design. The alarm itself is attached to pajamas in a variety of ways, for example, by being placed into a pocket sewn into the child's pajamas or pinned to them. Two wire leads extending from the alarm are attached (e.g., by small alligator clamps) on or near the pajama bottoms. When the child wets during the night, absorption of urine by the pajamas completes an electrical circuit between the two wire leads and activates the alarm. A variety of stimuli is available for use with the pajama devices including buzzing, ringing, vibrating, and lighting as well as a variety of volumes. A recent paper described an informal assessment of a variety of devices yielding a range from 85–110 db (Mellon & Houts, 2006). Several alarms currently available, including vendor information, website, and prices, are listed in Table 6.

Table 6
Representative Sample of Bedwetting Alarms with 2009 Prices:

Dr-Sleeper by Anzacare
www.dri-sleeper.com
$69.50 standard–$152.00 wireless

Nytone Enuretic Alarm
www.nytone.com
$75.00

Malem Bedwetting Alarm Starter Kit
www.BedwettingStore.com
$115.00-$164.95

Nite Train'r
www.nitetrain-r.com
$69.00

Potty Pager (vibrate only)
www.pottypager.com
$75.00

Wet-Stop3 by PottyMD
www.wet-stop.com
$50.00

3.3.1.3   Child- and Parent-Focused Methods

There are many ways to use the alarms, but the primary distinguishing factor involves the roles played by child and parent in alarm-based treatment. In child-focused methods, the alarm awakens the child, who independently manages the accident him- or herself (e.g., toileting, changing clothing and bedding). The most recent example of child-focused methods involves use of a vibrating (rather than sound producing) urine alarm (Ruckstuhl, 2003). In the parent-focused method the alarm awakens or alerts the parent, who in turn awakens the child, and they jointly manage the accident. The treatment procedures vary across published accounts and manuals, but generally include full arousal, going to the bathroom to complete (or attempt) urination, changing bedding and pajamas, resetting the alarm, and going back to bed. Parent-focused methods are obviously dependent on the saliency of the alarm stimulus. With the bed device, wire leads can be extended to the parent's bedroom. For the pajama device, either a very loud alarm or periodic checking is necessary to alert parents to the occurrence of an accident. Although the principles of learning would suggest that the earlier parents respond to accidents (e.g., immediately after the alarm sounds) the better the outcome, no data are available to support this position. After prescribing an alarm program, it is always best to supply a descriptive handout. A representative handout that can be used for a child and parent is provided in the Appendix.

3.3.2   Mechanisms of Action

The mechanism of action in alarm treatment was initially described as classical conditioning, with the alarm as the unconditioned stimulus, bladder distention as the conditioned stimulus, and waking as the conditioned response (Mowrer & Mowrer, 1938). More recent literature emphasizes a negative reinforcement or avoidance process (Friman, 2008; Ruckstuhl, 2003) whereby the child increases sensory awareness to urinary need and exercises physiological responses (e.g., contraction of the pelvic floor muscles) that prevent or quickly terminate urination and thereby avoid setting off the alarm (Mellon, Scott, Haynes, Schmidt, & Houts, 1997). Cures are obtained slowly, and, during the first few weeks of alarm use, the child often awakens only after having completed voided. The aversive properties of the alarm, however, gradually strengthen responses that lead to its avoidance. These responses are the same as those used regularly by continent persons who forestall urination after detecting a urinary urge that cannot be acted upon in the short term.

For example, at the moment the captain of a commercial airliner announces to passengers that the "fasten seatbelt sign" will soon be illuminated prior to landing, many passengers look toward the lavatories to determine whether they can be successfully used. A long line precludes their use, leaving the urinary urge unsatisfied and unsatisfiable in the short term. For most passengers in this situation, a collection of preventive physiological responses is initiated, typically with little or no conscious awareness. The responses include strategically using pelvic floor muscles to elevate the bladder neck and complete a "dry" Kegel exercise (see section on Kegel exercises). Successful execution of the responses typically allows the afflicted passengers to complete the flight, gather luggage, and in many instances get to their desired location prior to finding a bathroom and urinating successfully. In other words, the responses extend the passengers' capacity for continence well beyond the emergence of urinary urge. Although not definitive, the body of literature on the physiology of urination and alarm-based conditioning of continence suggests that children in alarm-based conditioning programs for enuresis learn to use the same type of responses to produce nocturnal continence (Kegel, 1951; Mellon et al., 1997; Muellner, 1960, 1961; Vincent, 1974).

3.3.3 Efficacy

Reports of controlled comparative trials show that the alarm-based treatment is superior to drug treatment and other nondrug methods such as retention control training (see below). In fact, numerous reviews of the literature show its success rate is higher and relapse rate lower than any other method – ranging as high as 80% for success and as low as 15% for relapse (Friman, 2008; Mellon & McGrath, 2000). One problem with interpreting the review literature on alarm treatment is that supplemental components are often added to improve effectiveness, resulting in the treatment "packages" described below. Additionally, there is very little research on child-based methods; we found only one study, and it reported an almost 50% success rate (Ruckstuhl, 2003).

Controlled comparative trials show that the alarm-based treatment is superior to drug treatment and other nondrug methods

3.3.4 Variations and Combinations of Methods

In principle, the urine alarm can be used as an effective single component treatment. In practice it is almost always part of a collection of methods or of a "treatment package." The oldest, best-known, and empirically supported treatment package is called dry bed training (DBT; Azrin, Sneed, & Foxx, 1974). Initially evaluated for use with a group of adults with profound mental retardation, it has since been systematically replicated numerous times across child populations. In addition to the bed alarm, the initial program components included overlearning, intensive cleanliness (responsibility) training, intensive positive practice (of alternatives to wetting), hourly awakenings, close monitoring, and rewards for success. In subsequent iterations, the stringency of the waking schedule was reduced and retention control training was added (e.g., Bollard & Nettlebeck, 1982).

Other similar programs were also developed; the best known and empirically supported one is the full spectrum home training (FSHT; Houts & Liebert, 1985; Houts, Liebert, & Padawer, 1983). FSHT includes the alarm, cleanliness training, retention control training, and overlearning. There are multiple variations now available. Component analyses have been conducted on both major programs, and the findings show that the alarm is the critical element, and that the probability of success increases as the number of additional components are added (Bollard & Nettlebeck, 1982; Houts, Peterson, & Whelan, 1986). The following section describes a broad range of optional components, starting with those that either have independent empirical support or that have been part of programs with empirical support. The section then describes a series of components that have weaker empirical support and are sometimes used alone or along with some of the components discussed previously.

3.3.5   Empirically Supported Components of Conventional Programs

3.3.5.1   Retention control training (RCT)

The emergence of retention control training followed the observation that many enuretic children had reduced functional bladder capacity

The emergence of RCT followed the observation that many enuretic children had reduced functional bladder capacity (Muellner, 1960, 1961; Starfield, 1967). RCT expands functional bladder capacity by requiring children to drink extra fluids (e.g., 16 ounces of water or juice) and delay urination as long as possible to increase the volume of their diurnal urinations and expand the interval between urges to urinate at night. Parents are instructed to establish a regular time for RCT each day and conclude the training at least a few hours before bedtime. Progress can be assessed by monitoring the amount of time the child is able to delay urination and/or the volume of urine they are able to produce in a single urination. Either or both can be incorporated into a game context wherein children earn rewards for progress. RCT is successful in as many as 50% of cases (Starfield & Mellits, 1968).

3.3.5.2   Kegel/Stream Interruption Exercises

Stream interruption exercises can often help in the treatment of enuresis

Kegel exercises involve purposeful manipulation of the muscles necessary to prematurely terminate urination or contraction of the muscles of the pelvic floor (Kegel, 1951; Muellner, 1960). Originally developed for stress and post-partum incontinence in women (Kegel), a version of these exercises – stream interruption – has been used in enuresis treatment packages for years (Friman, 2008). For children, stream interruption requires initiating and terminating urine flow at least once a day during a urinary episode. The use of stream interruption exercises in the treatment of enuresis is logical from a physiological perspective, because terminating an actual or impending urinary episode involves the same muscle systems. A major study of Kegel exercises showed their regular practice eliminated accidents in 47 of 79 children with diurnal enuresis.

3.3.5.3   Waking Schedule

This treatment component involves waking enuretic children and guiding them to the bathroom for urination. Results obtained are attributed to a change in arousal, increased access to the reinforcing properties of dry nights (Bollard & Nettlebeck, 1982), and urinary urge in lighter stages of sleep (Scharf & Jennings, 1988). In a representative study using a staggered waking schedule, four of nine children reduced their accidents to less than twice a week, suggesting that a waking schedule may improve (but is unlikely to cure) enuresis (Creer & Davis, 1975). The early use of waking schedules typically required full awakening, often with sessions that occurred in the middle of the night (e.g., Azrin et al., 1974; Creer & Davis, 1975), but two subsequent studies showed that partial awakening (e.g., Rolider & Van Houten, 1986; Rolider, Van Houten, & Chlebowski, 1984) or conducting waking sessions just before the parent's normal bedtime (Bollard & Nettlebeck, 1982) was just as effective. In additional, evaluations of the role of the waking schedule, when included in DBT and FSHT, produced contrasting findings: When used in DBT, Bollard and Nettlebeck (1982) showed that a combination of only the alarm and a waking schedule produced positive results, comparable to the use

When waking schedules are used, we recommend against the middle-of-the-night version of the entire treatment package. However, when used in FSHT, Whelan and Houts (1990) found no differences between groups that received FSHT with and without a waking schedule. In light of the existing, somewhat conflicting, research results, when waking schedules are to be used, we recommend against waking in the middle of the night in favor the less stringent approaches described previously (e.g., Friman, 2008).

3.3.5.4   Overlearning
An adjunct related to RCT involves overlearning. Like the RCT procedure, this method requires children to drink extra fluids – but just prior to bedtime. The overlearning procedure is a deliberate attempt to produce multiple accidents nightly through increased fluid intake and thereby increase learning trials in which the accidents instigate an alarm-based consequence. Overlearning is an adjunctive strategy only, used primarily to increase the maintenance of treatment effects already achieved through the urine alarm. Thus, it should not be initiated until a state of dryness has been reached (e.g., 7 dry nights; Houts & Liebert, 1985).

3.3.5.5   Cleanliness Training
Some form of effort directed toward returning soiled beds, bed clothing, and pajamas to a presoiled state is a standard part of DBT (Azrin et al., 1974), FSHT (Houts & Liebert, 1985; Houts, Peterson, & Liebert, 1984), and "package"-type treatments. It has, however, not been evaluated independently of other components, so that the extent of its contribution to outcome is unknown. Yet its contribution to the logic of treatment and consonance with conventional household expectations suggests its status as a treatment component is probably justified.

3.3.5.6   Reward systems
Contingent rewards alone are unlikely to cure enuresis, but they are an important component of DBT (Azrin et al., 1974). They have been included in many multiple component treatment programs since its development and are routinely recommended in papers describing effective treatment (e.g., Christophersen & Friman, 2004; Friman, 2008). With the current state of the literature, it is impossible to determine their independent role in treatment. One plausible possibility is that they sustain the enuretic child's motivation to participate in treatment, especially when the system reinforces success in small steps. If dry nights are initially infrequent and motivation begins to wane, decreases in the size of the urine stain can be used as the criteria for earning a reward. In the initial report of this method, tracing paper was laid over the spot and the number of 1-inch squares contained within the spot was counted (Ruckstuhl, 2003).

An example of an often used reward system involves the dot-to-dot method described in Table 7. Using this method allows parents to reward their incontinent child for small amounts of progress made on the way to continence and, thus, potentially to increase motivation.

Obviously, there are numerous combinations and variations on the empirically supported treatments for enuresis. As indicated previously, those with the most supportive evidence are DBT (Azrin et al., 1974) and FSHT (Houts & Liebert, 1985; Houts et al., 1984). However, virtually every enuresis expert

Table 7
The Dot to Dot Reward System for Treatment of Enuresis

1. Identify an item the child wants and parents are willing to buy.
2. Draw (or have drawn) a picture of it using dots. If the item is expensive, use lots of dots. A rule of thumb is $.50–$1 per dot.
3. Have the parents post the drawing with the child's name on top in a clearly visible place (e.g., refrigerator).
4. For every dry night, accident-free day, or episode with evidence of a smaller accident, have the parents permit the child to connect one dot.
5. When all of the dots have been connected, have the parents purchase and supply the item – immediately.
6. Warn parents that connected dots can never be taken away.
7. To make the program more interesting, add in a secondary system involving a grab bag.
8. Have parents write out small rewards on 25-50 slips of paper. These could include small manipulable toys, candy (if permitted), small amounts of money (dime, quarter), time withmother or father, extra bedtime, small privileges, etc. One or two large rewards could also be added (e.g., $5, select movie for family). Place all the slips in a bag (or bowl or hat).
9. Make every third dot in the dot to dot program bigger than the rest.
10. When the child reaches a big dot, have parents allow him or her to retrieve one slip from the grab bag and immediately deliver whatever is on the slip.
11. Have the parents return the slip to the bag.

Table 8
Summary of Moffat's (1997) Urine Alarm Procedures

1. Contract with parent and child for a 3-month trial.
2. Have the child keep a diary, starting at least 2 weeks before the first visit. It should include the number of wet nights, the number of accidents per night, and the size of the stain.
3. Require that the parent be part of the alarm system (because many children do wake to the alarm on their own initially but after a few weeks of parental help they gradually do).
4. Encourage detection of, emphasis on, and reward for arousal.
5. See the parent and child at least every 3 weeks initially.
6. Use three signs of improvement: decreased frequency of wet nights, number of episodes per night, and size of urine stain.
7. Continue until the child achieves 14 consecutive dry nights (no alarm sound – even for a spot of urine).
8. After the initial goal is achieved, use overlearning – either at least 16 ounces of fluid before bed or gradual 2-ounce increments, increasing as each step is mastered, until 16 ounces is reached.
9. Continue overlearning until the child achieves 14 consecutive dry nights.
10. Relapses can be re-treated successfully in the same manner, in many cases.

Adapted with permission from Moffatt, M. E. (1997). Nocturnal enuresis: A review of the efficacy of treatments and practical advice for clinicians. *Journal of Developmental and Behavioral Pediatrics, 18,* 49-56.

has developed their own variation on treatment or combination of treatment components and many of these are available on line (e.g., Collins, http://www.soilingsolutions.com/drybed.htm retrieved May 7, 2009), in books (e.g., Schaefer, 1995), and in peer-reviewed journals (Moffatt, 1997). In Table 8, we provide one example of these derived from Moffatt's 1997 paper published in a major behavioral pediatric journal.

3.3.6   Additional Components with Less Empirical Support

3.3.6.1   Self-Monitoring

Self-monitoring provides data that can be used to evaluate progress; when used for that purpose, it does not appear to involve treatment. One simple method for monitoring accidents merely requires the child to record (e.g., on a calendar) whether the previous night was wet or dry. A more complex and more sensitive method involves the size of spot measure as described previously (Ruckstuhl, 2003). In addition to its supplying data, however, the literature on self-monitoring shows that it has reactive properties and thus can actually be considered a treatment component. The direction of the change self-monitoring brings about is determined by the valence of the behaviors monitored (e.g., Nelson, 1977). Because afflicted children view nocturnal wetting negatively, self-monitoring can reduce the frequency of bedwetting.

> The literature on self-monitoring shows it has reactive properties and is actually an important treatment component

3.3.6.2   Hypnotism

A major obstacle to appraising hypnotism from an evidence-based perspective is the difficulty in operationally defining what hypnotism actually is. Here we consider it hyper-relaxation brought about by an arousal-reducing verbal interaction between child and therapist, the end result of which is an increase in instructional control or susceptibility to suggestion. Once the relaxed state has been achieved, the therapist makes a number of suggestions pertaining to continence. In the best-known study using hypnosis for treatment of enuresis, 31 of 40 subjects became fully continent (Olness, 1975). A subsequent independent study reported full continence in 20 of 28 bedwetting participants (Stanton, 1979). The results of the two studies, although remarkable, were reported more than 25 years ago, and full independent replications have not been reported since. Additionally, studies attempting to determine the additive role of hypnosis to treatment packages have produced inconsistent results (e.g., Banerjee, Srivastay, & Palan, 1993; Edwards & Van Der Spuy, 1985).

3.3.6.3   Paired Associations

Paired association involves pairing Kegel exercises (stream interruption) with the urine alarm in a reward-based program. In a typical scenario, a tape recording of the urine alarm sounding at strategically placed temporal intervals is taken into the bathroom by the child and played as urination proceeds. At each sounding of the alarm on the tape, the child stops urine flow. The number of starts and stops are then included in part of a reward-based interaction between child and parent. The paired association procedure has yet to be evaluated, but some basic literature supports at least its potential effectiveness. For example, sleeping persons can make discriminations between stimuli on the basis of meaningfulness and prior training (Oswald, Taylor, & Treisman, 1960), and the probability of a correct discrimination is significantly improved through contingent reinforcement (Zung & Wilson, 1961). Thus, reinforcing a relationship between stream interruption and the alarm while the child is awake may increase the probability that the child will interrupt urination in response to the alarm while asleep.

3.3.7   Medication

Physicians prescribe drug therapy for enuresis more often than they prescribe any other treatment (e.g., Vogel, Young, & Primack, 1996). Because of the necessity of physician involvement in enuresis, the widespread use of drug therapy by physicians – and the dominating influence of the biobehavioral model of enuresis – it is likely that medication will often become part of the treatment regimen. We therefore briefly discuss here the two most commonly prescribed types of medications, antidepressants and antidiuretics.

3.3.7.1   Tricyclic antidepressants

Historically, tricyclic antidepressants were the drugs of choice for the treatment of enuresis, and imipramine was the most frequently prescribed drug of this class (Blackwell & Currah, 1973). However, the mechanism by which imipramine reduces bed wetting has never been conclusively established. In doses between 25 and 75 mg, given at bedtime, imipramine has produced initial reductions in wetting in substantial numbers of enuretic children, often within the first week of treatment. However, enuresis usually recurs when the tricyclic therapeutic agents are withdrawn, so that the permanent cure rate is only about 25%.

3.3.7.2   Antidiuretics

Norgaard and colleagues reported on a small number of enuretic children who had abnormal circadian patterns of ADH (e.g., Norgaard et al., 1985). As a result of these reports, desmopressin (DDAVP, an analog of ADH, rapidly became a popular treatment for enuresis, displacing the tricyclics as the most prescribed treatment. DDAVP concentrates urine, thereby decreasing urine volume and intravesical pressure, which makes the physiological dynamics that precede urination less probable and nocturnal continence more probable. Conventionally recommended dosages are 10–20 micrograms taken at bedtime.

Research on the effectiveness of DDAVP has yielded mixed results with success in some studies (e.g., Dimson, 1986) but not in others (Scharf & Jennings, 1988). A recent review indicated that fewer than 25% of children become dry on the drug (a much larger percentage show some improvement), and similar to tricyclics its effects appear to last only as long as the drug is taken and are less likely to occur in younger children or children who have frequent accidents (Moffat, Harlos, Kirshen, & Burd, 1993). Nonetheless, its treatment effects, when they do occur, are as immediate as those produced by imipramine. Because DDAVP was initially thought to produce fewer side effects (e.g., Dimson, 1986; Norgaard et al., 1985), it became preferable to imipramine as an adjunct to treatment. Moreover, a review of the relevant literature suggested including DDAVP with alarm-based treatment had the potential to boost the already high success obtained by the alarm to 100% (Mellon & McGrath, 2000). That optimistic perspective, however, recently shifted toward pessimism due to the discovery of potentially fatal side effects resulting from regular dosing – see the section on DDAVP below.

3.3.8 Problems in Carrying Out the Treatments

3.3.8.1 Alarm-Based Treatment
The primary problem in carrying out alarm-based treatment involves prema-ture termination, a form of medical noncompliance that has been reported to be as high as 48% (Turner, Young, & Rachman, 1970). The causal role of sev-eral psychological variables has been explored (e.g., parental attitudes toward enuresis, self-esteem), but no causal relation has been established. Alarm-based treatment does require considerable effort and patience, and although no research on the role of effort in premature termination has been published, there is a substantial literature showing the reductive effect effort has on medical compliance in general (e.g., Friman & Poling, 1995). As indicated above, alarm-based treatments are substantially more effective than drug-based treatments – but they are also substantially more difficult to administer and maintain. Despite frequent recommendations against using medication as the primary treatment for enuresis, physicians prescribe medications far more often that they do behavioral methods, and parental preferences support that practice (Fergusson et al., 1986; Rauber & Maroncelli, 1984). In sum, a major obstacle to overcome in the prescription of alarm-based treatment is the rela-tive difficulty it takes to use and the time it takes to work, especially relative to other treatments such as medication.

> **The primary problem in carrying out treatment involves premature termination**

3.3.8.2 Medication-Based Treatment
The primary problems with the two dominant medication-based treatments, imipramine and DDAVP, are the temporary results and the risk of serious side effects. For example, imipramine is well tolerated in prescribed dosages, but is toxic when these dosages are exceeded. In the 1970s it was the most com-mon cause of fatal ingestion by children under the age of 5 (Cronin, Khalil, & Little, 1979). Although most victims of imipramine poisoning took excessive amounts of the medication by accident, some took it deliberately in a tragically futile attempt to expedite progress in their treatment (e.g., Herson, Schmitt, & Rumack, 1979). The triad of symptoms associated with excessive use includes coma, convulsions, and cardiac disturbances. Because of the risk of serious side effects on the one hand, and the benign nature of enuresis on the other, it is a medication with a problematic risk/benefit ratio. Due to its limited effective-ness, temporary effects, and risk factors, it should be used only as an *adjunct* to other treatment – and for children in unstable family environments it should not be used at all!

> **The primary problems associated with the two dominant medication based treatments, imipramine and DDAVP, are temporary results and the risk of harmful side effects**

The benefits of DDAVP, when they do occur, are also temporary (see com-ments above), and it too is associated with serious side effects. For example, recent reports by the US Food and Drug Administration (FDA) have alerted the public to potential dangers posed by DDAVP, especially when delivered in its most popular form – intranasal spray. Specifically, some persons taking DDAVP are at risk of developing a sodium deficiency in their blood, called hyponatremia, which can result in seizures and death. Children treated with the *intranasal* form of DDAVP for enuresis are particularly susceptible to severe hyponatremia and seizures. Therefore, the Food and Drug Administration made three relevant rulings: First, intranasal DDAVP is contraindicated for the treatment of enuresis and should not be used in hyponatremic patients or patients with a history of hyponatremia. Second, treatment of enuresis with DDAVP in tablet form should be suspended during acute illnesses that might lead to fluid and/or electrolyte imbalance. Third, DDAVP should always be used cautiously in patients at risk for water intoxication with hyponatremia (US FDA, 2007). These rulings are likely to have a notable impact on interventions for enuresis, given the pervasiveness of the problem and the popularity of DDAVP as a treatment. Psychologists may be able to successfully capitalize on the resulting gap in treatment options available to medical providers by offering evidence-based biobehavioral alternatives.

3.4   Case Vignette: Nocturnal Enuresis

History. Fred, a 10-year-old boy, was living at home with his natural parents and two younger sisters, ages 6 and 8, with whom he got along well, with the exception of some teasing because of his bedwetting. He was in the fifth grade and did well in school both behaviorally and academically. He presented at an Outpatient Behavioral Pediatric and Family Services Clinic with complaints of chronic bedwetting. His medical, psychiatric, educational, and developmental histories were unremarkable. His parents were both professionals and worked full-time jobs outside the home. Both parents were college educated. The clinical history indicated that, beyond the current concern, there were no other behavioral complaints. Fred had been daytime trained since the age of 3 and had yet to have an accident-free night. His social life was somewhat constrained because he had had urinary accidents on sleepovers and at camp. He had worn a pull up to bed up until age 8 when he requested to be allowed to go to bed in pajamas.

The referring psychologist requested a physical examination to be conducted by his primary-care doctor, which ruled out medical causes of the nocturnal enuresis. A family history revealed that his mother had been nocturnally incontinent until the age of 9, and an uncle on his father's side had been nocturnally incontinent until the age of 11. A developmental screening was negative for delays, and a psychological screening was negative for significant behavioral and emotional problems. As indicated, however, there was mounting evidence of social problems stemming from his chronic incontinence. Specifically, he refused to attend camp and denied requests from friends to spend the night. He also discontinued the practice of inviting friends to spend the night at his house. An assessment of parental attitudes toward enuresis indicated tolerance on the part of both parents, although it was somewhat more limited in the father than in the mother. Both parents and child were highly motivated to seek treatment.

Assessment. The assessment of Fred's accidents indicated that they occurred once or twice a night. His parents intermittently woke him to visit the bathroom, and if an accident had already occurred, they changed his bedding and required that he change his pajamas. He never changed his bedding or pajamas on his own without prompting from parents, and his mother routinely changed his bedding during the day. He provided no assistance with the laundry of his wet pajamas and bedding. No consequences were applied for accidents, and because he had not yet had a dry night, parental response for success was moot. During the assessment period, Fred assented to measurement of his daytime urine output and use of a common household measuring cup for six urinations showed an average of 4 ounces, which was quite small for a child his age. He urinated an average of 8–10 times a day.

Case Conceptualization. Fred's urinary accidents met the diagnostic criteria from the DSM-IV for Primary Monosymptomatic Nocturnal Enuresis. As is typical of most cases of enuresis, it appeared to be inherited, with potential genetic lines of transmission on both sides of the family. The case was not complicated by extraneous psychosocial factors, nor was it yet complicated by comorbid behavioral problems. But there was evidence of a gradually shrinking social life, and Fred rarely slept away from his home. There was also clear evidence of reduced functional bladder capacity and overly frequent daytime urinations. The average volume for a continent child his age should be between 10 and 14 ounces, and his was around 4 ounces. Additionally, 4-6 urinations a day should be sufficient for a 10-year-old boy.

Treatment. Consistent with the description of treatment for enuresis in this paper, the primary component of treatment selected for Fred was the urine alarm – one that attached to his pajamas. As discussed previously, the effectiveness of treatment increases as additional components are added to a treatment plan. These are best selected collaboratively by therapist, child, and parents, as was done in this case. Fred and his parents selected the following additional components:

1. A motivational system involving the dot-to-dot program described earlier in the paper, wherein Fred would earn a cherished videogame when his drawing was complete.
2. Responsibility training requiring Fred to bring stained bed clothing and pajamas to the basement laundry room and to remake his own bed after an accident.
3. A two-week period of overlearning during which Fred drank extra fluids before bed and during the day on weekends.
4. Dry Kegel exercises conducted several times during the day and at least one start/stop exercise conducted while urinating each day.
5. RCT on the weekends.
6. A self-monitoring system involving Fred recording wet and dry nights on a calendar supplied by the therapist.
7. A weekly parent monitoring system involving sizing urine stains on either Saturday or Sunday night.
8. A visualization exercise requiring Fred to imagine waking up in a dry bed in the morning.
9. Tablet-based DDAVP to be supplied as needed whenever Fred spent the night away from home.

Outcome. Fred's therapist monitored progress by interviewing the parents and Fred himself, inspecting Fred's self-monitoring calendar, and reviewing progress on the dot-to-dot drawing and variations in the urine spot measurement. During a 2-week pretreatment baseline, Fred wet the bed nightly and the urine spots were very large because of the overlearning component of treatment that was imposed during baseline. In the first week following treatment, Fred's frequency of accidents sank to 5 nights a week and continued to fall for 5 continuous weeks, at which point accidents ceased altogether. At that point the major components of the program were phased out. In the 6 months following, Fred had two accidents, both of which involved small amounts of urine. At the 1-year follow-up, Fred had not had an accident for at least 6 months.

4

Diurnal Enuresis

4.1 Description

4.1.1 Terminology and Definition

The vast majority of cases of enuresis are nocturnal and, correspondingly, most of the literature on enuresis is devoted to the nocturnal type. Nonetheless, enuresis cases that involve a diurnal component are a notable concern, especially in late preschool and early elementary school. Although the pertinent literature is small, it strongly suggests that diurnal enuresis is a justifiable cause of concern for afflicted children, their caretakers, and teachers. Along with the risk of secondary psychological problems (discussed under section 4.1.5 Comorbidities below), there are public health concerns associated with daytime wetting. For example, the increase in the prevalence of infectious disease (e.g., hepatitis, infectious diarrhea) seen in daycare settings and preschools over the past few decades has been partially attributed to the spread of bacteria through child incontinence (Berk & Friman, 1990; Hadler & McFarland, 1986; Pickering, Bartlett, & Woodward, 1986).

4.1.2 Epidemiology

Because of the limited research on diurnal enuresis, virtually all aspects of it are less well understood than parallel aspects of nocturnal enuresis. This is true even for something as straightforward as prevalence. One reason is that although the DSM-IV diagnostic criteria are clear, they may be too exclusive. For example, a 5-year-old who wets his bed 1 or 2 times a week poses no serious problem for himself or his family. But a 4-year-old who wets his pants at preschool 1 or 2 times a week may pose problems for himself, his teachers, and his parents. Yet the DSM criteria would capture the former and not the latter case. Prevalence estimates for the two ages also vary widely. Most papers on enuresis as a general topic supply epidemiological information only for the nocturnal version (e.g., American Academy of Child and Adolescent Psychiatry, 2004). The most widely cited published estimate of troublesome day time wetting between the ages of 5 (the cutoff age for the DSM criteria) and 7 years, whether it strictly diurnal or mixed, is .5%–2% of children (Blomfield & Douglas, 1956). A slight majority of these cases are girls, as distinct from nocturnal enuresis, where a clear majority of cases are boys.

Because of the limited research on diurnal enuresis, virtually all aspects of it are less well understood than parallel aspects of nocturnal enuresis

4.1.3   Course and Prognosis

For most cases
of non medical
diurnal enuresis, the
prognosis is very
good, especially with
treatment

The prognosis is very good for most cases of nonmedical diurnal enuresis, , especially with treatment. Yet even without treatment there is a high rate of remission, and functional chronic daytime wetting in middle school, high school, and beyond that is rare and usually associated with developmental disabilities, major psychiatric conditions, postpartum complications, and old age. However, one recent paper estimated that one-fifth of cases persist into adulthood (Bernard-Bonnin, 2000), though it supplied no empirical support for the estimate.

4.1.4   Differential Diagnosis

As with nocturnal enuresis, there are multiple physiopathological causes of diurnal enuresis, and they can be grouped into medical and functional categories. The literature subdivides the medical category into infection, disease, and anatomical abnormalities; but with the exception of sleep apnea, the members of these categories essentially mirror the medical causes of nocturnal enuresis. Although these medical conditions may all require behavioral interventions as part of a comprehensive treatment plan, the initial and primary management is medical.

The literature also subdivides the functional category, although there is much less agreement as to its categories. The following list is representative of the diverse literature: excessive urinary deferral, vaginal reflux, labial fusion, daytime frequency syndrome, giggle incontinence, stress incontinence, emotional stress, and the unstable bladder of childhood (Bauer et al., 1980; Bernard-Bonnin, 2000; Meadow, 1990).

Some children simply
hold their urine until
they can do so no
longer and, thereby,
raise the risk of
accidents

Urinary deferral. Some children simply hold their urine until they can do so no longer and thereby increase the risk of accidents. Why they do so has not been actually determined, but it could be related to anxiety. It could also involve intense concentration (e.g., videogames) or participation (e.g., baseball) in other activities. In addition to raising the risk of accidents, extreme urinary deferral can also raise the risk of urinary tract infection and urinary reflux.

Vaginal reflux. Some girls present with urinary incontinence because they do not open their labia sufficiently to allow optimal urine flow. As a result, some urine is retained in the vagina and it is released involuntarily (through gravity) when they stand up. Girls who are obese or who sit deep into the toilet seat while urinating are particularly at risk.

Daytime frequency syndrome. Some toilet-trained children are afflicted by the sudden onset of excessively frequent urinary urges (e.g., every 5–10 minutes). The average duration of the syndrome is 2–3 months, and it typically terminates almost as suddenly as it emerges. It is more frequent in boys at an average age of 5 years; its etiology has not been established.

Giggle incontinence. This condition is almost solely confined to girls and its presentation is sporadic. The most typical scenario involves an instance of intense or prolonged giggling (thus its name) that rapidly triggers the urinary urge process and results in bladder emptying.

Physical stress incontinence. This condition results from the inadvertent mismanagement of the pelvic floor muscles (see the previous section on *Physiology of Urination*), resulting in the relaxation of urinary sphincter muscles and bladder emptying. The most typical causes are high physical exertion, sneezing, or coughing.

Emotional stress incontinence. This condition can involve isolated events brought on by extremely stressful stimulation. Examples are frequently used in movies to depict the saliency, immediacy, and extremity of a threat to a character's life. The Academy award-winning movie *The Unforgiven* includes a memorable example. The condition can also persist if the afflicted child is exposed to persistent stressful stimulation. Children subject to chronic physical or sexual abuse are at risk for this condition. However, the emotional stress that leads to this type of incontinence need not be aversive. The anticipation of highly pleasurable events (e.g., parties, trips, special occasions) can also induce emotional stress incontinence in children.

> **Children subject to chronic physical or sexual abuse are at risk for emotional stress incontinence**

The unstable bladder of childhood. This is a "wastebasket" term for a variety of conditions that result in incontinence – in fact it includes most of the conditions listed above (Bauer et al., 1980). Among the various conditions subsumed under this category, however, there is one that has not yet been mentioned: bladders that have been variously referred to as hypersensitive, hyperreflexive, or hyperresponsive (Bauer et al., 1980; Berg, 1979; Meadow, 1990). Afflicted children can volitionally void urine but are also subject to premature bladder contractions and nonvolitional voiding. The condition is associated with maturational delay (as with most causes of urinary incontinence) and affects mostly girls (for reasons unknown).

Idiopathic (i.e., "garden variety") diurnal incontinence. Obviously, the functional category of diurnal enuresis – the category that includes nonmedical causes – is large and diverse. However, all of the various subcategories are united by one feature: Each is responsive to a combination of health education and behavioral intervention. Although medication is also occasionally used for some types (e.g., unstable bladder of childhood), educating parents and afflicted children about the condition and supplying treatment recommendations drawn from those described in the Treatment section 4.3 below is the primary approach. To simplify the discussion, from this point on we subsume all of the functional categories into one: idiopathic diurnal enuresis.

> **The cardinal variable in the biobehavioral approach to idiopathic diurnal enuresis is awareness**

The cardinal variable in the biobehavioral approach to idiopathic diurnal enuresis is awareness – awareness of bladder distension and incipient or actual bladder neck descent (see section on Physiology of the Bladder). This distension and/or descent gives rise to postural changes and limb movements suggestive of urinary urgency. The function of these movements appears to be maintenance of bladder neck ascent. For example, when children scissor their legs or compress their thighs the movements produce upward pressure in the perineal region that lifts the bladder neck and forestalls urination. These movements, and their function, are paradoxical, however, in that children are often unaware of them and of their urinary urgency. So, when parents advise their children to go the bathroom, based on observation of these movements, the children may appear surprised and unaware of the need. Routine aspects of parental teaching can be applied to help the child make the necessary connections, initially between body movements and need – and ultimately between bladder contraction and need – and thereby enable the child to complete or forestall urination based on a plan.

A major variable inhibiting attainment of the awareness needed for continence is reduced functional bladder capacity (Fielding, 1982; Friman & Jones, 1998). This limitation is due primarily to either functional capacity variables (as with nocturnal enuresis) or partial emptying. Children with these problems have poor control over their pelvic floor musculature and/or immature bladders (oversensitive to filling). Behavior problems (e.g., noncompliance) may also play a role in the failure to attain daytime continence.

Another inhibitory variable that inhibits awareness of wetness rather than urinary urge is the prolonged wearing of absorptive undergarments (e.g., pull-ups). A popular commercial and cultural trend toward increased usage of these garments appears to promote convenience over continence by postponing (e.g., in young children) or forgoing (e.g., in the handicapped or elderly) continence training (Blum, Taubman, & Nemeth, 2009; Lancaster, 1990). Some preliminary evidence suggests that this trend could actually perpetuate incontinence (e.g., Tarbox, Williams, & Friman, 2004).

> **A major variable inhibiting the attainment of awareness needed for continence is reduced functional bladder capacity**
>
> **Another inhibitory variable that inhibits awareness of wetness rather than urinary urge is the prolonged wearing of absorptive undergarments**

4.1.5   Comorbidities

The scientific literature on diurnal enuresis and psychological comorbidity is composed primarily of descriptive findings from uncontrolled examinations conducted more than 20 years ago. Because diurnal enuresis is much more likely than nocturnal enuresis to be detected by persons outside the afflicted child's family, thus increasing the possibility of growing costs such as social distance and reduced social standing, it is a much greater psychological risk factor. For this reason, it is surprising that comorbidity has received so little scientific attention, especially in contrast with the abundant attention paid to nocturnal enuresis and comorbidity. This scientific gap reflects in part the more general differential between scientific interest in nocturnal versus diurnal enuresis. The scientific literature on the former is vast, while the literature on the latter is scant.

The minimal interest in diurnal enuresis and even more minimal interest in comorbidity may have led to a secondary reason for the gap, one that is more responsible for maintaining than causing it: A tendency to generalize the research on nocturnal enuresis to diurnal enuresis suffuses the literature, and this is particularly true with respect to comorbidities or secondary psychological problems. This tendency is evident in at least two ways. The first is the most common: subsuming diurnal enuresis into a more general discussion of nocturnal enuresis and addressing diurnal wetting only obliquely – if at all. This tendency is even evident in some (e.g., Friman, 2008), but fortunately not all (e.g., Christophersen & Friman, 2004), of our own papers on enuresis. The second involves direct discussion of diurnal enuresis including descriptions of secondary psychological problems but with references only to papers on nocturnal enuresis (e.g., Coury, 2002). We found only three actual data-based papers: two peer reviewed (Berg, Fielding, & Meadow, 1977; Halliday, Meadow, & Berg, 1987) and the other an unpublished doctoral dissertation (Fielding, 1978). Collectively, these papers report an increase in antisocial behaviors in day-wetting children compared to night-wetting and nonwetting children, but all three were provided by essentially the same group of researchers. Subsequent reviews of the literature concluding that day-wetting enuretic children exhibit an increase in psychiatric problems were also from the same group (e.g., Berg, 1979; Meadow, 1990). Clearly, an independent replication would be helpful, although the fact that the data-based papers were published more 20 years ago – with essentially no attempts at direct or systematic replication – may mean that continence researchers consider the question settled. If so, a persuasive case can be made that it should be revisited.

Another compelling reason for the further study of comorbidity is that enuresis of any sort also constitute a large source of stress in the life of afflicted children, ranking along with divorce and parental fights (Van Tijen, Messer, & Namdar, 1998) – and there is a persuasive basis for viewing the diurnal version as more stressful than nocturnal. For example, there is a much increased likelihood of detection: Diurnal accidents can happen in any domain of an afflicted child's social life, and the visual and olfactory cues generated by accidents heighten the risk of social detection. Evasive action could reduce the likelihood of detection, but diurnal enuresis is often accompanied by limited self-awareness (Fielding, 1982). Accidents are thus often initially detected by someone else. If that someone is a sympathetic parent, the social cost for the child is minimal. But not all parents are sympathetic or understanding: Incontinence is a leading cause of child abuse (Finn, 2005; Helfer & Kempe, 1976). Additionally, not all of the adults who detect accidents will be the parents; some will be teachers and not all of them will be sympathetic or understanding. Teacher reluctance to allow children to use the bathroom during class hours was recently widely discussed and debated in the media (MacDonald, 2007).

Finally, not all of the persons who detect accidents will be adults; some will be peers or other older or younger children. The socially aversive aspect of peer detection is revealed by research on the greatest fears of childhood – fear of urinary accidents at school ranks just after fear of losing a parent and going blind (Allantoic, King, & Fray, 1989). The high level of this fear is unsurprising in light of the literature on child reaction to differences in their peers. It shows that children are often highly critical of developmental and behavioral differences in their peers, especially if those differences are viewed as maladaptive and potentially under the control of the child who exhibits them (e.g., Sigelman & Begley, 1987). Epidemiological research shows that most children have achieved full continence by the age of 4 (Berk & Friman, 1990), so that any urinary accidents in older children detected by peers are likely to be viewed negatively, ostracism being a real possibility. The extent of this concern is also reflected in the extent to which parents and their nocturnally enuretic children are willing to forgo important socializing events such as camp, sleepovers, and overnight trips with nonfamily members to avoid detection of nighttime accidents. In sum, although evidence in the literature is scant, there is good reason to view diurnal enuresis as a potential contributor to other comorbid problems in the lives of afflicted children. Fresh research on the question is needed to determine the nature and the extent of the problems.

Enuresis of any sort is a major source of stress in the life of afflicted children

Incontinence is a leading cause of child abuse

By the age of 4 most children have achieved full continence

4.1.6   Diagnostic Procedures and Documentation

The diagnostic procedures for diurnal enuresis are very similar to those used for nocturnal enuresis except that they involve checking clothing rather than bedding. The frequency, location, and approximate volume of accidents should be documented. The most frequently used method for accomplishing this task involves "dry pants checks." There are actually two functions for the checks, one for assessment and one for treatment. The assessment function involves determining the presence and size of urinary accidents. The treatment function involves setting the occasion for a parent to deliver a reward for dryness or corrective steps for accident. The intervals between checks can range from every 5 minutes to once a day. We recommend beginning with hourly checks and reducing the frequency once success has been achieved.

A less invasive measurement system involves having parents check their child's clothing once it has been removed for bed. This type of monitoring should be employed for assessment only; it should not initiate a treatment response because the time between the response and the accident may be so large that the child may not be able to form helpful associations. In either form of measurement, exact accident volumes are difficult to establish, though knowledge of exact volumes is not truly critical. Rather, it is merely necessary to determine whether a child's accidents involve dribbling or full bladder emptying. A final diagnostic procedure involves determining functional bladder capacity. Although not necessary in all cases, if a child's urination pattern seems excessively frequent, assessing FBC reveals whether it is low and, if so, set the occasion for including urine-retention exercises in treatment. Methods for assessing FBC and using urine retention are described the Nocturnal Enuresis section above.

4.2   Theories and Models of Diurnal Enuresis

As with all aspects of diurnal enuresis, there is a dearth of literature on differential theoretical models, especially compared with the literature on nocturnal enuresis. This dearth has dramatically simplified the theoretical picture: There are essentially two models, biobehavioral and medical. The former involves all of the components of the biobehavioral model of nocturnal enuresis except sleep dynamics;. the latter involves all of the differential diagnoses that have a medical dimension except sleep apnea.

4.3   Treatment for Diurnal Enuresis

4.3.1   Methods of Treatment, Mechanisms of Action, and Efficacy

4.3.1.1   Alarm-Based Treatment

There are few published studies describing effective biobehavioral treatment of diurnal enuresis in typically developing children, and the most prominent of these did not appear until the 1980s – which is puzzling because the studies with the best results employed the urine alarm (see description below). As noted previously, the effectiveness of the urine alarm for nocturnal enuresis

There are few published studies describing effective biobehavioral treatment of diurnal enuresis was demonstrated in the 1930s (e.g., Mowrer & Mowrer, 1938). Why it took almost 50 years to initiate major tests of the alarm for diurnal enuresis is unknown and, to our knowledge, not even discussed in the literature. One plausible possibility is that alarm-based treatment for daywetters had to await the invention of an alarm that attached to clothing rather than bedding. Clothing alarms created a day-based treatment alternative. The initial patent application for an alarm that could be worn on clothing was in 1970 (Caldwell, 1970), and it was quickly followed by several descriptive reports and case studies describing its potential for toilet training young children and persons with severe disabilities (e.g., Azrin, Bugle, & O'Brien, 1971). Its possibilities for treating diurnal enuresis in typically developing children were not explored experimentally until almost 20 years later (Halliday et al., 1987).

Perhaps investigators viewed diurnal enuresis as qualitatively different than nocturnal enuresis and thus not necessarily responsive to treatments shown to be effective for the nocturnal type. This view is not illogical. Nocturnal enuresis is not under volitional control whereas daytime wetting is. The primary reason for use of an alarm in nocturnal cases was that the afflicted children were asleep during the accidents, which is clearly not the case with daywetters. Therefore, its potential utility was not as evident. Additionally, some treatments shown to be effective for nocturnal enuresis were shown to be ineffective for diurnal enuresis. For example, urine retention training, a method shown to be successful with nocturnal enuresis (e.g., Starfield & Mellits, 1968), was unsuccessful when used on a group of daywetting children (Fielding, 1978; Fielding, Berg, & Bell, 1978).

Nonetheless, some investigators apparently began to see some functional similarities between daytime and nighttime wetters. For example, although daywetters are awake, they do not appear to be fully aware of urinary urge and, occasionally, even urinary accidents, and they also sometimes seem unmotivated to change (Fielding, 1982; Van Laecke et al., 2006). Therefore, treatments involving combinations of cueing and motivation were attempted. For example, a controlled single-case study showed that a cueing system combined with a reward program eliminated diurnal urinary accidents in a 19-year-old girl (Luiselli, 1987). Clinicians also began using the urine alarm as a cueing and consequence-based treatment, the Halliday et al. (1987) evaluation mentioned previously being the initial experimental report of its success. The study randomly assigned 44 children to two groups, in one of which the alarm went off randomly and in the other of which it went off immediately following an accident. Two-thirds of the children in both groups became dry, and there was no significant difference between groups. Consistent with the findings from Luiselli (1987), these results suggest that, when used with diurnal enuresis, the alarm may work as a cueing system as much as it does as a consequence.

Although daywetters are awake, they do not appear to be fully aware of their urge to urinate

The Halliday et al. (1987) study was systematically replicated in a controlled case study of a 15-year-old girl with diurnal enuresis. Pretreatment assessments revealed accidents occurred only at home, never in school, thus suggesting her wetting may have been responsive to social attention. Therefore, the alarm was used at home in contingent program wherein it sounded whenever she had an accident. Immediately following implementation of treatment, complete continence was attained and maintained at long-term follow-up (Friman & Vollmer, 1995).

A larger more recent retrospective study also systematically replicated the results of Halliday et al. (1987). The records of 63 children whose daytime wetting was treated with the urine alarm were examined, revealing that two-thirds of the children achieved full dryness or substantial improvement (Van Laecke et al., 2006).

A modest amount of empirical evidence supports the use of the urine alarm

In sum, although late in arriving on the diurnal enuresis scene, a modest amount of empirical evidence supporting the use of the urine alarm has now been published. Each of the existing three studies has its limitations, however, and even when these studies are considered as a group, their collective findings are merely suggestive, not definitive. Nonetheless, with one exception (mentioned below), alarm-based treatment is the only biobehavioral approach to diurnal enuresis with group-based empirical support. Furthermore, recent advances in the technology of urine alarms could enhance their potential as a primary treatment for diurnal enuresis. A number of alarmmakers now provide alarms that vibrate rather than emit noise, resulting in private but not public detection of accidents, a feature that could enhance the overall acceptability of the alarm as a treatment.

4.3.1.2   Kegel exercises

There is a discrepancy in the amount of research conducted on diurnal versus nocturnal enuresis

The one additional biobehavioral treatment for diurnal enuresis with empirical support, albeit only from one study, involves the practice of Kegel exercises. This study, also discussed in the treatment portion of the section on nocturnal enuresis above, reported that training 79 daywetting children to practice Kegel exercises at least 3 times a day eliminated accidents in 44 and substantively reduced them in another 9 (Schneider, King, & Surwitt, 1994).

Obviously, there is a discrepancy in the amount of research conducted on diurnal versus nocturnal enuresis. The former is tiny, especially when compared with the latter, which is vast (e.g., Friman, 2008). As discussed in the section on comorbidity, the public dimension of daytime accidents, and the resulting detrimental effect their detection can have on social distance, relations, and standing, would seem to supply more urgency for research on effective treatment. In the absence of clear empirically supported options, most medical practitioners – the professionals most likely to initially encounter daywetters – have proceeded with a variety of medical interventions (e.g., invasive bladder "rehabilitation," inpatient biofeedback treatment), none of which has much empirical support. Despite this gap in the literature, to assist the practitioner below we recommend a combination of components for initial treatment. The combination has not been empirically evaluated. but rather is composed of individual components that have. It is inexpensive and minimally invasive, especially compared with the other options described.

4.3.2   Variations and Combinations of Methods

Representative Multicomponent Treatment

In contrast to contemporary literature on treatment of nocturnal enuresis, which is abundantly populated by empirical analyses of multicomponent treatments (e.g., Azrin et al., 1974; Houts et al., 1983), we found no empirical evaluations of multicomponent approaches to diurnal enuresis in typically developing children. There are some case studies of multicomponent treatments for diurnal enuresis in persons with developmental disabilities (e.g., Azrin & Foxx, 1971); but the target problem in these cases involved urinary incontinence that is more accurately viewed as resulting from incomplete or absent toilet training than from what we have characterized as diurnal enuresis. Additionally, the intensity of the methods used with persons with developmental disabilities make them unsuitable –and almost certainly unacceptable – for programs for typically developing young children with diurnal enuresis. In the interest of serving the readers, however, we supply a description of a representative multicomponent approach to treatment beginning with the initial encounter.

As with the initial encounter with cases of nocturnal enuresis, the medical causes of diurnal enuresis need first to be identified and medically treated or ruled out. Major psychological complications also need to be addressed prior to any treatment regimen. All forms of punishment implicit and explicit should be eliminated. Treatment should focus on known causes of urinary accidents that can be addressed with health education and biobehavioral treatment methods. Some cases may be resolved with only two components: education about the condition and some condition-specific health recommendations. For example, a toileting schedule consistent with healthful urination patterns may be all that is needed for children who excessively defer urination. Teaching parents to teach their girls afflicted with vaginal reflux to more fully open the labia during urination can solve that problem. Girls who release urine during laughter can be taught to exhibit their response to humorous episodes in a more demure fashion. Unmotivated children can be placed on a motivational program. Providing counseling about stress management could resolve incontinence in children whose wetting accidents are associated with emotional stress.

All forms of punishment, implicit or explicit, should be eliminated

For children whose urinary incontinence more likely results from maturational factors – and that is the majority of cases – the three likely causes are reduced awareness of urge, insufficient use of pelvic floor musculature, and low motivation. For these children several components may be necessary for optimal outcomes. Treatment could begin with an assessment of the timing of urinations, accidents, and successes throughout the day. A toileting schedule linked to the outcome of the assessment could be established. Kegel exercises could be taught and subsequently used to increase pelvic floor involvement. A clothing-based urine alarm could be used to increase awareness of urinary urge and to cue the need for pelvic floor muscle manipulation. Because of its reduced social saliency, the vibrating alarm may be preferable to the sound-based alarm (Ruckstuhl, 2003). It is difficult to imagine cases that would *not* benefit from a motivational component. However, the construction of the program is important: Prior to contact with professionals, parents may be inclined to offer large incentives (e.g., bicycle, recreational electronics) for full continence. Unfortunately, such offers can effectively have a detrimental effect on motivation. When full continence is the criteria for the incentive, a single accident can reset the program to its starting point, thus actually adding existing costs to the problem for the child. To be optimally effective, incentive programs should provide children with the experience of success for small steps toward continence. For example, children on the dot-to-dot program mentioned previously could be allowed to connect a dot for merely having a fully continent morning. They would not earn their full reward until the dots were all connected, but they would have the experience of moving toward that goal by meeting a small objective.

It is difficult to imagine cases of incontinence that would not benefit from a motivational component

On weekends, the overlearning component described in the treatment section on nocturnal enuresis could be added to increase learning trials. For children at risk for accidents in school, a classroom pass program can be used, in which the child is given a pass that allows them to leave class to use the bathroom without penalty. To discourage abuse of the pass program, the child can be provided small incentives for unused passes at the end of the school day. Finally, responsibility training could be included to lessen parental labor and heighten child motivation to improve.

We recommend including as many treatment components as parents are willing to implement and the child is willing to accept

As discussed previously, multicomponent treatments drawn from these various components have yet to be empirically evaluated for diurnal enuresis. However, two likely core components, Kegel exercises and the urine alarm, proved to be moderately successful. The other components are typically included in treatments for nocturnal enuresis, and evaluations of those programs have shown that, in alarm-based programs, as the number of components increase so too does the chance of success. Thus, for optimal treatment, we recommend including as many components related to the type of diurnal enuresis a child has that parents are willing to implement and the child is willing to accept. Table 9 provides the clinician with a summary of a representative multicomponent treatment for diurnal enuresis.

Table 9
Summary of Representative Multicomponent Treatment for Diurnal Enuresis

- Physical exam to rule out medical causes.
- Address psychological complications (e.g., impaired instructional controls skills).
- Eliminate all forms of punishment, direct and indirect.
- Focus treatment on specific causes of the condition if known.
- Supply health education about the cause (e.g., excessive urinary referral results in "urgency" accidents and potential health problems, overenthusiastic laughter can cause accidents).
- Supply behavioral treatment specific to the cause if known (e.g., prompted toilet visits for excessive urinary deferral, demure laughter for giggle incontinence).
- For maturational cases (with no known specific cause), assess the timing of urinations over several days).
- Establish a toileting schedule based on the results of the assessment.
- Teach and subsequently prompt start-stop exercises (Kegel); require the child to practice at least once a day.
- Purchase and use a vibrating urine alarm – but only for home use.
- Establish a monitoring system for accidents and accident-free periods.
- Establish and use a reward system for accident-free periods (e.g., dot-to-dot reward system).
- On weekends, use the over learning procedure – but only at home.
- For in-school programming, use the bathroom pass.

4.3.3　Problems in Carrying Out the Treatments

As with nocturnal enuresis, the best results for treatment of diurnal enuresis have been attained with the urine alarm. The primary problem with its use is noncompliance. However, although there is a small body of research exploring the reasons for noncompliance with treatment for nocturnal enuresis, we found none exploring the reasons for noncompliance with treatment for diurnal enuresis. A plausible guess would be the effort involved increases in which often produce decreases in the rate of desirable behavior (e.g., Friman & Poling, 1995). As described above, the optimal treatment regimen includes multiple components, each of which involves parental and child effort. An additional problem involves the potential stigma of the urine alarm: Social detection of urinary accidents is a potentially highly aversive event for incontinent children, especially if they are attending school. Use of a sound-based alarm substantially heightens the probability that accidents will be detected by others. There are at least two ways to address this problem.

> The best results for treatment of diurnal enuresis have been attained with the urine alarm. The primary problem with using it is noncompliance

The first involves implementing the alarm component of treatment only at home (e.g., at night and on weekends). The second involves use of the vibrating urine alarm, though it is not completely soundless and thus too increases the risk of social detection, although not to the degree that the sound-based alarm does. Nonetheless, because of children's sensitivity to risk of social awareness of their condition, alarm-based treatment, whether with sound or the vibrating device, should not be conducted outside the home without clear evidence of child agreement.

4.4　Case Vignette: Diurnal Enuresis

History. Sam, a 6-year-old boy, lived at home with his natural parents and older brother, Tom, age 12. He was in the first grade. His teacher had no complaints about his academic progress, but she was concerned about emerging socially withdrawn behavior and a pattern of diurnal incontinence that she felt was at least partially responsible for the withdrawal. He presented at an Outpatient Behavioral Pediatric and Family Services Clinic for treatment of the daytime wetting problems. His medical, psychiatric, educational, and developmental histories were unremarkable. His father was a plumber and his mother held a part-time job as a sales clerk. Both parents had high-school educations. The clinical history indicated that with the exception of the incontinence and the emerging social problems, there were no other behavioral complaints. He had been toilet trained successfully at the age of 3 but began having urinary accidents when he entered kindergarten. He was continent at night. His parents managed his wetting accidents using absorptive undergarments (pull-ups), but following the advice of friends, they had made a small number of attempts to address the wetting with reward systems, scheduling, and removal of the absorptive undergarments. The results of their efforts were unfortunately unsuccessful and resulted in two accidents at school that were detected by his teacher and his peers. Subsequently, he returned to wearing the absorptive undergarments which he was using at the time of the referral.

The referring psychologist requested a physical examination to be conducted by his primary-care physician, which ruled out medical causes of the diurnal wetting. A family history revealed that an uncle on his mother's side had been a bedwetter, though the parents could not recollect daytime wetting problems in their own histories nor in the histories of other close relatives. A developmental screening was negative for delays, and a psychological screening was negative for significant behavioral and emotional problems. However, the screening did indicate psychometric evidence of the social withdrawal noted by his teacher. In addition to avoiding others on the playground, he refused to attend camp and expressed little interest in having friends visit him at his home. He was also reluctant to visit friends at their homes, and at the time of the referral, the parents and the boy could not identify any classmate or neighbor as a close friend. An assessment of parental attitudes toward the wetting indicated tolerance on the mother's part and intolerance on the father's part. The father believed that Sam was inattentive and mildly lazy about his toileting responsibilities. His mother believed that he simply could not help it. Both the mother and Sam were highly motivated to pursue treatment, but the father did not participate in any clinic visits. The mother reported that the father was supportive but unable to find the time to come to the clinic.

Assessment. Assessment of Sam's urinary patterns indicated that he was completely continent at night. Because he wore a pull-up, the frequency of his accidents during the day was impossible to determine on school days, but he came home wet at least 4 days a week. To estimate accident frequency during the assessment period, he did not wear pull-ups on the weekends, and the frequency across 4 weekend days was 1.25 accidents a day. Parental response to the accidents varied depending on the parent. The mother tended to note neutrally that he had had an accident, guide him to the bathroom, encourage him to attempt to urinate, and then change his clothing. His father was more firm and sometimes more critical, and supplied much less assistance. He would merely note that his boy had an accident, comment critically, and tell him to go change his clothes. The mother also assessed his urinary output using a glass measurement container on three occasions, and the result indicated an average of approximately 3.5 ounces per measure. She also estimated that he urinated an average of 7–9 times a day when he was not in his pull-up.

Case Conceptualization. Sam's urinary accidents met criteria from the DSM-IV for Primary Diurnal Enuresis. It also fit criteria for a secondary classification because he had had a period of complete continence lasting longer than 6 months. There was modest evidence supporting its being an inherited condition. There was also evidence that the chronic accidents were producing an increasingly growing detrimental effect on Sam's social life, largely because he had had accidents at school, and peers and teachers had detected them. There was also evidence of substantially reduced functional bladder capacity and overly frequent daytime urinations. There was no evidence that the onset of the accidents was occasioned by a trauma or chronic encounter with serious distressful events. These facts supported the view that it was an idiopathic ("garden variety") case of diurnal enuresis.

Treatment. The core component for treatment for Sam's incontinence while at home was the vibrating urine alarm. But, because of the potential for enhanced detection at school by classmates, it was not used there. Because of the elevated motivation of Sam and his mother, multiple components were assembled to create a treatment package. These included the following:

1. A motivational system involving the dot-to-dot program mentioned earlier. The ultimate reward he selected was a basketball.

2. A toileting schedule was implemented both at home and school. At school, he was directed to use the toilet between two classes in the morning and two classes in the afternoon.

3. A toileting pass program was implemented at school which allowed him to leave class whenever he felt the urge to urinate, at which point he would surrender his pass. For each unused pass, he was provided one sticker, and the accumulation of five stickers allowed him to withdraw one small reward from a classroom reward bag.

4. The use of pull-ups was discontinued at school.

5. Wet Kegel exercises were conducted 2–3 times a week at home.

6. RCT was conducted on the weekends.

7. A self-monitoring system with which Sam recorded accident-free days on a specially constructed chart at home was implemented.

8. A modification of the father's typical response to accidents was requested and, according to the mother, actually realized. The father was simply asked to provide a neutral response to accidents and avoid any form of criticism.

9. Although Sam was too young to assist with laundry, he was required to bring his own soiled clothing to the laundry basket whenever he had an accident.

Outcome. Sam's therapist monitored his progress through telephone contacts with the mother and periodic clinic visits. He would either inquire about or actually inspect the self-monitoring calendar and the dot-to-dot drawing. During a 2-week baseline, Sam was wet almost every day and slightly more frequently on the weekends. Immediately following the implementation of treatment, accidents at school stopped but continued periodically on the weekends. By week 4 he was completely accident-free, at which point the use of the alarm was discontinued. When he completed his dot-to-dot program and earned his reward, the system was discontinued as was the calendar-based monitoring system. At week 7 all major components of the program were discontinued. At the 6-month follow up, Sam had not had an accident for at least 4 months.

4.5   Summary and Conclusions

History has not been kind to children with enuresis. They have suffered at the hands of their parents, peers, friends, neighbors, and even professionals sought by parents to help with the problem. Although it is true that attitudes toward enuresis as well as parental and professional approaches to it have improved substantially overtime, especially in comparison with the approaches from antiquity, there is still much progress to be made. For example, despite abundant evidence of the problematic side effects from medication, including accidental death, in standard practice medical treatment still trumps psychological treatment. However, as documented in this book, although there are

History has not been kind to children with enuresis

multiple evidence-based approaches to enuresis, they are infrequently sought or prescribed, at least in comparison to other approaches that lack supportive evidence. For example, fluid restriction is almost universally recommended by professionals and used by parents – and yet no supportive evidence has ever been supplied to support this approach to the treatment of enuresis.

Evidence-based treatment for enuresis always requires some time and trouble

Effort is almost certainly one of the major obstacles to use of evidence-based approaches. For example, medication and fluid restriction require almost no effort, while the treatment programs with the most supportive evidence include multiple components and require considerable effort from both parents and children. Thus, the former methods are much more likely to be used than the latter – at least when begun in the absence of evidence-based professional guidance. At present there is no easy way to solve this problem. Evidence-based treatment for enuresis simply always require some time and trouble. Nonetheless, there is solid scientific support for use of just one treatment component, the urine alarm, whether the problem is nocturnal or diurnal. Although the alarm involves more effort than medication or fluid restriction, it involves substantially less effort than the standard multicomponent treatment programs. Thus alarm-only programs appear to provide a middle ground between medical or efficient nonevidence-based programs on the one hand, and major multicomponent treatments on the other.

Although virtually all children with elimination problems eventually attain their goal, their progress can be substantially expedited through strategic use of evidence-based approaches

A practitioner can improve the life of an enuretic child substantially even if alarm-based treatment is not suitable at the time of treatment. For example, Kegel exercises require little effort to teach and practice and have some evidence-based support for both nocturnal and diurnal enuresis. RCT requires more effort than Kegel exercises but less than the alarm, and they too have been shown to be effective (e.g., Starfield & Mellits, 1968). There are also some nondirect approaches to treatment that can benefit afflicted children. For example, as described previously, enuresis is routinely misinterpreted. The provider can employ health education to correct misimpressions. Home remedy motivational systems often produce either no results or results that actually reduce motivation (e.g., offering a large and very desirable reward, but only for full continence). Practitioners can revise the systems and supply information needed for effective design of new systems. Protective undergarments are readily available, yet extended use can interfere with toileting progress. Practitioners can schedule reduced use in a way that complements the requirements of effective treatment. More generally, practitioners can induce a sense of optimism into a home-based context that is likely to be marked by at least some and, perhaps a great deal, of pessimism. Full continence is a cornerstone of civilized, socialized development across cultures. Because of a slight genetic variation in a surprisingly large number of families, many children are very late in achieving this highly desirable goal. Although virtually all will ultimately attain the goal, their progress can be substantially expedited through strategic use of evidence-based approaches to enuresis in its various forms.

5

General Conclusion

Because of the physiological components involved, many child and family psychologists may be inclined to refer incontinent children to "specialists" for assessment and treatment. As strongly emphasized in this book, it is paramount that all psychologists first refer incontinent children to a physician for a physical examination to rule out (or in) physiopathological processes known to cause fecal or urinary incontinence. However, one of the primary intentions of this book was to provide psychologists with the clinical tools necessary to implement an initial treatment plan and possibly avoid the need for consultation with experts. Although it is true that consultation with experts is a standard component of competent clinical practice, *consultation with this book is*, in a sense, *consultation with experts*. The two authors have assessed and treated more than a thousand incontinent children. We are painfully aware of the long dark history of child incontinence, and we view the evidence-based practices described in this book as opportunities for psychologists to help incontinent children realize much brighter futures than with those available to most incontinent children throughout history. We do not view our book as an inaugural foray into childhood incontinence. Publications on defecation and urination practices have multiplied tremendously in the past few decades. For example, a very influential social scientist and bestselling author recently wrote, "The last decade has seen an explosion of books about poop" (Gilbert, 2005, p. 215). Something similar could also be accurately said about pee (sic). Nonetheless, our book does not merely add one publication to this growing body of literature; rather, it extends that body by distinguishing fact from fancy in the assessment and treatment of childhood incontinence and emphasizes approaches that are supported by hard science. In conclusion, we hope child clinicians will use this book to guide their practice with incontinent children, and that at least some, possibly many, will consider attempting initial treatment where they previously would have been inclined to refer. In so doing, they will have added to the growing ranks of clinicians whose approach to childhood incontinence is guided by scientific evidence rather than whim, unsubstantiated theory, or antiquated convention.

The last decade has seen an explosion of books about poop; the same could be said about pee

6

Further Reading

The interested reader is referred to the following article for a comprehensive review of the empirically supported treatments for constipation and encopresis: McGrath, M.L., Mellon, M.W. and Murphy, L. (2000). Empirically supported treatments in pediatric psychology: Constipation and encopresis. *Journal of Pediatric Psychology, 25,* 225–254.

The October 2001 issue of *Journal of the American Academy of Child and Adolescent Psychiatry* was devoted to an extensive review of the research literature on enuresis and encopresis.

Christophersen, E. R., & Mortweet, S. L. (2001). *Treatments that work with children: Empirically supported strategies for managing childhood problems.* Washington, DC: APA.

Schmitt, B. D. (1984). Nocturnal enuresis. *Primary Care, 11,* 485–495.

Schmitt, B. D. (1984). Encopresis. *Primary Care, 11,* 497–511.

Schonwald, A. D., & Sheldon, G. G. (2006). *The pocket idiot's guide to potty training problems.* Indianapolis, IN: Penguin.

7

References

Achenbach, T. M. (1991). *Manual for the child behavior checklist: 4–18 and 1991 profile*. Burlington, VT: University of Vermont, Department of Psychiatry.

Allantoic, T. H., King, N. J., & Fray, R. (1989). Fears in children and adolescents: Reliability and generalizability across gender, age, and nationality. *Behavior Research and Therapy, 27,* 19–26.

American Academy of Child and Adolescent Psychiatry. (2004). Practice parameter for the children and adolescence with enuresis. *Journal of the American Academy of Child and Adolescent Psychiatry, 43,* 1540–1550.

American Psychiatric Association. (1994). *Diagnostic and statistical manual of mental disorders* (4th ed.). Washington, DC: Author.

Arnell, H., Hjalmas, K., Jagervall, M., Lackgren, G., Stenberg, A., Bengtsson, B. et al. (1997). The genetics of primary nocturnal enuresis: inheritance and suggestion of a second major gene on chromosome 12 q. *Journal of Medical Genetics, 34,* 360–365.

Azrin, N. H., & Bugle, C., & O'Brien, F. (1971). Behavioral engineering: Two apparatuses for toilet training retarded children. *Journal of Applied Behavior Analysis, 4,* 249–253.

Azrin, N. H., & Foxx, R. M. (1971). A rapid method of toilet training for the institutionalized retarded. *Journal of Applied Behavior Analysis, 4,* 89–99.

Azrin, N. H., Sneed, T. J., & Foxx, R. M. (1974). Dry-bed training: Rapid elimination of childhood enuresis. *Behavior Research & Therapy, 12,* 147–156.

Baeyens, D., Roeyers, H., Hoeheke, P., Verte, S., Van Hoecke, E., & Walle, J. V. (2004). Attention deficit/hyperactivity disorder in children with nocturnal enuresis. *Journal of Urology, 171,* 2576–2579.

Baker, S. S., Liptak, G. S., Colletti, R. B., Croffie, J. M., DiLorenzo, C., Ector, W., & Nurko, S. (1999). Constipation in infants and children: evaluation and treatment. *Journal of Pediatric Gastroenterology and Nutrition, 29,* 612–626.

Bakwin, H. (1973). The genetics of enuresis. In I. Kolvin, R. C. MacKeith, & S. R. Meadow (Eds.), *Bladder control and enuresis* (pp. 73–78). Philadelphia, PA: Lippincott.

Banerjee, S., Srivastav, A., & Palan, B. (1993). Hypnosis and self hypnosis in the management of nocturnal enuresis: A comparative study with imipramine therapy. *American Journal of Clinical Hypnosis, 36,* 113–119.

Barkley, R. A. (1997). *ADHD and the nature of self control.* New York: Guilford.

Barr, R. G., Levine, M. D., Wilkinson, R. H., & Mulvihill, D. (1979). Chronic and occult stool retention: A clinical tool for its evaluation in school-aged children. *Clinical Pediatrics, 18,* 674–686.

Bauer, S. B., Retik, A. B., Colodny, A. H., Hallett, M., Khoshbin, S., & Dyro, F. M. (1980). The unstable bladder of childhood. *Urologic Clinics of North America, 7,* 321–336.

Berg, I. (1979). Day wetting children. *Journal of Child Psychology and Psychiatry, 20,* 167–173.

Berg, I., Fielding, D., & Meadow, R. (1977). Psychiatric disturbance, urgency, and bacteriuria in children with day and night wetting. *Archives of Diseases of Children, 52,* 651–657.

Berk, L. B., & Friman, P. C. (1990). Epidemiological aspects of toilet training. *Clinical Pediatrics, 29,* 278–282.

Bernard-Bonnin, A. C. (2000). Diurnal enuresis in childhood. *Canadian Family Physician, 46,* 1109–1115.

Bingley, P. J., Williams, A. J. K., Norcross, A. J., Unsworth, D. J., Lock. R. J., Ness, A. R., & Jones, R. W. (2004). Undiagnosed celiac disease at age seven: Population-based prospective birth cohort study. *British Medical Journal, 328*, 322–323.

Bishop, W. P. (2001). Miracle laxative? *Journal of Pediatric Gastroenterology and Nutrition, 32*, 514–515.

Blackwell, B., & Currah, J. (1973). The psychopharmacology of nocturnal enuresis. In I. Kolvin, R. C. MacKeith, & S. R. Meadow (Eds.), *Bladder control and enuresis* (pp. 231–257). Philadelphia: Lippincott.

Blomfield, J. M., & Douglas, J. W. B. (1956). Bedwetting: Prevalence among children 4 to 7 years old. *Lancet, I,* 850–852.

Blum, N., Taubman, B., & Nemeth, N. (2004). Why is toilet training occurring at older ages? A study of factors associate with later training. *The Journal of Pediatrics, 145,* 107–111.

Blum, N. J., Taubman, B., & Osborne, M. L. (1997). Behavioral characteristics of children with stool toileting refusal. *Pediatrics, 99,* 50–53.

Bollard, J., & Nettlebeck, T. (1982). A component analysis of dry-bed training for treatment of bed-wetting. *Behavior Research & Therapy, 20,* 383–390.

Borowitz, S. M., Cox, D. J., Tam, A., Ritterband, L. M., Sutphen, J. L., & Penberthy, J. K. (2003). Precipitants of constipation during early childhood. *Journal of the American Board of Family Practice, 16*, 213–218.

Borowitz, S. M., Cox, D. J., Sutphen, S. L., & Kovatchev, B. (2002). Treatment of childhood encopresis: A randomized trial comparing three treatment protocols. *Journal of Pediatric Gastroenterology and Nutrition, 34*, 378–384.

Brody, J. E. (1992, January 29). Personal health: silence on fecal incontinence is harmful; From 1 to 2 percent of children over 4 have the problem. *New York Times*, pp. B8.

Browne, N. D. F. (1986). Some enuretic derivatives in an adult analysis. *International Journal of Psychoanalysis, 67,* 449–447.

Caldwell, J. W. (1970). Enuresis prevention training device (United States Patent # 3696357). Retrieved February 21, 2009 from http://www.freepatentsonline.com/3696357.html

Christophersen, E. R. (1982a). Behavioral pediatrics [whole issue]. *Pediatric Clinics of North America, 29.*

Christophersen, E. R. (1982b). Incorporating behavioral pediatrics into primary care. *Pediatric Clinics of North America, 29,* 261–296.

Christophersen, E. R. (1991). Toileting problems in children. *Pediatric Annals, 20,* 240–244.

Christophersen, E. R. (1994). *Pediatric compliance: A guide for the primary-care physician.* New York: Plenum.

Christophersen, E. R., & Friman, P. C. (2004). Elimination disorders. In R. Brown (Ed.), *Handbook of pediatric psychology in school settings* (pp. 467–488). Mahwah, NJ: Erlbaum.

Christophersen, E. R., & Mortweet, S. L. (2001). Diagnosis and management of encopresis. In E. R. Christophersen & S. L. Mortweet, *Treatments that work with children: Empirically supported strategies for managing childhood problems.* Washington, DC: APA.

The Constipation Guideline Committee of the North American Society for Pediatric Gastroenterology, Hepatology and Nutrition (NASPGHAN) (2006). Clinical Practice Guideline: Evaluation and treatment of constipation in infants and children: Recommendations of the North American Society for Pediatric Gastroenterology, Hepatology, and Nutrition. *Journal of Pediatric Gastroenterology and Nutrition, 43,* e1–e13.

Conners, C. K. (1969). A teacher rating scale for use in drug studies with children. *American Journal of Psychiatry, 126,* 884–888.

Coury, D. (2002). Developmental and behavioral pediatrics. In A. M. Rudolph, R. K. Kamei, & K. J. Overby (Eds.), *Rudolph fundamentals of pediatrics* (3rd ed., pp. 110–124). New York: McGraw-Hill.

Cox, D. J., Morris, J. B., Borowitz, S. M., & Sutphen, J. L. (2002). Psychological differences between children with and without chronic encopresis. *Journal of Pediatric Psychology, 27*, 585–591.

Creer, T. L., & Davis, M. H. (1975). Using a staggered waking procedure with enuretic children in an institutional setting. *Journal of Behavior Therapy & Experimental Psychiatry, 6,* 23–25.

Cronin, A. J., Khalil, R., & Little, T. M. (1979). Poisoning with antidepressants: An avoidable cause of childhood deaths. *British Medical Journal, 1,* 722.

Davidson, M. (1958). Constipation and fecal incontinence. *Pediatric Clinics of North America, 5,* 749–757.

Davidson, M., Kugler, M. M., & Bauer, C. H. (1963). Diagnosis and management in children with severe and protracted constipation and obstipation. *Journal of Pediatrics, 62,* 261–275.

DeLeon, G., & Mandell, W. (1966). A comparison of conditioning and psychotherapy in the treatment of functional enuresis. *Journal of Clinical Psychology, 22,* 326–330.

Dimson, S. B. (1986). DDAVP and urine osmolality in refractory enuresis. *Archives of Diseases in Children, 61,* 1104–1107.

Dwyer, J. T. (1995). Dietary fiber for children: How much? *Pediatrics, 96,* 1019–1022.

Edwards, S., & Van Der Spuy, H. (1985). Hypnotherapy as a treatment for enuresis. *Journal of Child Psychology and Psychiatry, 26,* 161–170.

Farrell, R. J., & Kelly, C. P. (2002). Current concepts: Celiac sprue. *New England Journal of Medicine, 346,* 180–188.

Fergusson, D. M., Horwood, L. J., & Shannon, F. T. (1986). Factors related to the age of attainment of nocturnal bladder control: An 8-year longitudinal study. *Pediatrics, 78,* 884–890.

Fielding, D. (1978). *An investigation of some factors influencing the classification and treatment of childhood enuresis with special reference to day time wetting.* Ph.D. Thesis, University of Leeds, UK.

Fielding, D. (1982). An analysis of the behavior of day- and night-wetting children: Toward a model of micturation control. *Behavior Research and Therapy, 20,* 49–60.

Fielding, D., Berg, D. M., & Bell, S. (1978). An observational study of postures and limb movements of children who wet by day and at night. *Developmental Medicine and Child Neurology, 20,* 453–461.

Finn, R. (2005). Clinic rounds. *Pediatric News, 39*(11), 43.

Forsythe, W., & Redmond, A. (1974). Enuresis and spontaneous cure rate study of 1129 enuretics. *Archives of Diseases in Children, 49,* 259–269.

Foxman B., Valdez R. B., & Brook, R. H. (1986). Childhood enuresis: Prevalence, perceived impact and prescribed treatments. *Pediatrics, 77,* 482–487.

Friman, P. C. (2008). Evidence based therapies for enuresis and encopresis. In R. G. Steele, T. D. Elkin, & M. C. Roberts (Eds.), *Handbook of evidence-based therapies for children and adolescents* (pp. 311–333). New York: Springer.

Friman, P. C., Handwerk, M. L., Swearer, S. M., McGinnis, C., & Warzak, W. J. (1998). Do children with primary nocturnal enuresis have clinically significant behavior problems? *Archives of Pediatrics and Adolescent Medicine, 152,* 537–539.

Friman, P. C., & Jones, K. M. (1998). Elimination disorders in children. In S. Watson, & F. Gresham (Eds.), *Handbook of child behavior therapy* (pp. 239–260). New York: Plenum.

Friman, P. C., & Vollmer, D. (1995). Successful use of the nocturnal urine alarm for diurnal enuresis. *Journal of Applied Behavior Analysis, 28,* 89–91.

Friman, P. C., Mathews, J. R., Finney, J. W., Christophersen, E. R., & Leibowitz, M. (1988). Do encopretic children have clinically significant behavior problems? *Pediatrics, 82,* 407–409.

Friman, P.C., & Poling, A. (1995). Life does not have to be so hard: Basic findings and applied implications from research on response effort/force. *Journal of Applied Behavior Analysis, 28,* 583–590.

Fritz, G. K., & Anders, T. F. (1979). Enuresis: The clinical application of an etiologically based system. *Child Psychiatry and Human Development, 10,* 103–111.

Gabel, S., Hegedus, A. M., Wald, A., Chandra, R., & Chiponis, D. (1986). Prevalence of behavior problems and mental health utilization among encopretic children: Implications for behavioral pediatrics. *Journal of Developmental and Behavioral Pediatrics, 7,* 293–297.

Gellis, S. S. (1994). Are enuretics Truly hard to arouse? *Pediatric Notes, 18,* 113.

Gilbert, D. (2005). *Stumbling on happiness.* New York: Random House.

Glicklich, L. B. (1951). An historical account of enuresis. *Pediatrics, 8,* 859–876.

Gross, R. T., & Dornbusch, S. M. (1983). Enuresis. In M. D. Levine, W. B. Carey, A. C. Crocker, & R. T. Gross (Eds.), *Developmental-behavioral pediatrics* (pp. 575–586). Philadelphia, PA: Saunders.

Hadler, S. C., & McFarland, L. (1986). Hepatitis in day care centers: Epidemiology and prevention. *Review of Infectious Disease, 8,* 548–557.

Halliday, S., Meadow, S. R., & Berg, I. (1987). Successful management of daytime enuresis using alarm procedures: A randomly controlled trial. *Archives of Diseases in Children, 62,* 132–137.

Helfer, R., & Kempe, C. H. (1976). *Child abuse and neglect.* Cambridge, MA: Ballinger.

Hellman, D. S., & Blackman, N. (1966) *Enuresis, firesetting and cruelty to animals: A triad predictive of adult crime. American Journal of Psychiatry, 122,* 1431–1435.

Herson, V. C., Schmitt, B. D., & Rumack, B. H. (1979). Magical thinking and imipramine poisoning in two school-aged children. *Journal of the American Medical Association, 241,* 1926–1927.

Houts, A. C. (1991). Nocturnal enuresis as a biobehavioral problem. *Behavior Therapy, 22,* 133–151.

Houts, A. C. (2000). Commentary: Treatments for enuresis: Criteria, mechanisms, and health care policy. *Journal of Pediatric Psychology, 25,* 219–224.

Houts, A. C., & Liebert, R. M. (1985). *Bedwetting: A guide for parents.* Springfield, IL: Thomas.

Houts, A. C., & Liebert, R. M., & Padawer, W. (1983). A delivery system for the treatment of primary enuresis. *Journal of Abnormal Child Psychology, 11,* 513–519.

Houts, A. C., Mellon, M. W., & Whelan, J. P. (1988). Use of dietary fiber and stimulus control to treat retentive encopresis: A multiple-baseline investigation. *Journal of Pediatric Psychology, 13,* 435–445.

Houts, A. C., Peterson, J. K., & Liebert, R. M. (1984). The effects of prior imipramine treatment on the results of conditioning therapy with NE. *Journal of Pediatric Psychology, 9,* 505–508.

Houts, A. C., Peterson, J. K., & Whelan, J. P. (1986). Prevention of relapse in Full-Spectrum Home Training for primary NE: A component analysis. *Behavior Therapy, 17,* 462–469.

Iacono, G., Cavataio, F., Montalto, G., Florena, A., Tumminello, M., Soresi, M., Notarbartolo, A., & Carroccio, A. (1998). Intolerance of cow's milk and chronic constipation in children. *New England Journal of Medicine, 339,* 1100–1104.

Ingebo, K. B., & Heyman, M. B. (1988). Polyethylene glycol-electrolyte solution for intestinal clearance in children with refractory encopresis. *American Journal of Diseases of Children, 142,* 340–342.

Joinson, C., Heron, J., Butler, U., & von Gontard, A. (2006). Psychological differences between children with and without soiling problems. *Pediatrics, 117,* 1575–1584.

Jose, C. J. (1981). Nocturnal enuresis caused by psychotropic drugs. *American Journal of Psychiatry, 138,* 1519.

Kaffman, M., & Elizur, E. (1977). Infants who become enuretics: A longitudinal study of 161 Kibbutz children. *Monographs of the Society for Research on Child Development, 42,* 2–12.

Kanner, L. (1972). *Child psychiatry.* Springfield, IL: Charles C. Thomas.

Kegel, A. H. (1951). Physiologic therapy for urinary stress incontinence. *Journal of the American Medical Association, 146,* 915–917.

Kendall, P .C., Flannery-Schroeder, E., Panichelli-Mindel, S. M., Southan-Gerow, M., Henin, A., & Warman, M. (1997). Therapy for youths with anxiety disorders: A second randomized clinical trial. Journal of Consulting and Clinical Psychology, 65, 366–380.

Key, D. W., Bloom, D. A., & Sanvordenker, J. (1992). Low-dose DDAVP in nocturnal enuresis. *Clinical Pediatrics, 32* 299–301.

Landman, G. B., Levine, M. D., & Rappaport, L. (1983). A study of treatment resistance among children referred for encopresis. *Clinical Pediatrics, 23,* 449–452.

Landman, G. B., & Rappaport, L. (1985). Pediatric management of severe treatment-resistant encopresis. *Development and Behavioral Pediatrics, 6*, 349–351.

Lancaster, M. M. (1990). Urinary incontinence: Aids for management. In R. C. Hanby, J. M. Turnball, L. D. Norman, & M. M. Lancaster (Eds.), *Alzheimer's disease: A handbook for caregivers* (pp. 108–115). St. Louis: Mosby.

Levine, M. D. (1975). Children with encopresis: A descriptive analysis. *Pediatrics, 56*, 412–416.

Levine, M. D. (1976). Children with encopresis: A study of treatment outcome. *Pediatrics, 56*, 845–852.

Levine, M. D. (1982). Encopresis: Its potentiation, evaluation, and alleviation. *Pediatric Clinics of North America, 29*, 315–330.

Levine, M. D. (1983). Encopresis. In M. D. Levine, W. B. Carey, & A. C. Crocker (Eds.), *Developmental-behavioral pediatrics* (2nd ed., pp. 389–397). Philadelphia: Saunders.

Loening-Baucke, V. A. (1994). Management of chronic constipation in infants and toddlers. *American Family Physician, 49*, 397–400, 403–406, 411–413.

Loening-Baucke, V. (1995). Biofeedback treatment for chronic constipation and encopresis in childhood: Long-term outcome. *Pediatrics, 96*, 105–110.

Loening-Baucke, V. A. (1996). Encopresis and soiling. *Pediatric Clinics of North America, 43*, 279–298.

Loening-Baucke, V. (2002). Polyethylene glycol without electrolytes for children with constipation and encopresis. *Journal of Pediatric Gastroenterology and Nutrition, 34*, 372–377.

Loening-Baucke, V. A., Cruikshank, B. M., & Savage, C. (1987). Defecation dynamics and behavior profiles in encopretic children. *Pediatrics, 80*, 672–679.

Luiselli, J. K. (1987). Secondary diurnal enuresis: Evaluation of a cueing and reinforcement interventions with a sensory impaired youth. *Journal of Mental Deficiency Research, 31*, 287–292.

Luxem, M. C., & Christophersen, E. R. (1999). Elimination disorders. In S. Netherton, D. Holmes, & C. E. Walker (Eds.) *Child and adolescent psychological disorders: A comprehensive textbook* (pp. 195–223). New York: Oxford.

Luxem, M. C., Christophersen, E. R., Purvis, P. C., & Baer, D. M. (1997). Behavioral-medical treatment of pediatric toileting refusal. *Journal of Developmental and Behavioral Pediatrics, 18*, 34–41.

MacDonald, G. J. (2007). Teachers can say no when kids have to go. *USATODAY.com*. Retrieved March 13, 2009 from, http://www.usatoday.com/news/education/2007-06-03-children-bathroom-breaks_N.htm

McGrath, M. L., Mellon, M. W., & Murphy, L. (2000). Empirically supported treatments in pediatric psychology: Constipation and encopresis. *Journal of Pediatric Psychology, 25*, 225–254.

McGuire, T., Rothenberg, M., & Tyler, D. (1983). Profound shock following interventions for chronic untreated stool retention. *Clinical Pediatrics, 23*, 459–461.

Meadow, S. R. (1990). Day wetting. *Pediatric Nephrology, 4*, 178–184.

Mellon, M. W., & Houts, A. C. (1995). Elimination disorders. In R. T. Ammerman & M. Hersen (Eds.), *Handbook of child behavior therapy in the psychiatric setting* (pp. 341–366). New York: John Wiley.

Mellon, M. W., & Houts, A. C. (2006). Nocturnal enuresis: Evidence based perspectives in etiology, assessment, and treatment. In J. E. Fisher & W. T. O'Donohue (Eds.,), *Practitioners guide to evidence-based psychotherapy* (pp. 432–441). New York: Springer.

Mellon, M. W., & McGrath, M. L. (2000). Empirically supported treatments in pediatric psychology: Nocturnal enuresis. *Journal of Pediatric Psychology, 25*, 193–214.

Mellon, M. W., Scott, M. A., Haynes, K. B., Schmidt, D. F., & Houts, A. C. (1997). *EMG recording of pelvic floor conditioning in nocturnal enuresis during urine alarm treatment: A preliminary study*. Paper presentation at the Sixth Florida Conference on Child Health Psychology, University of Florida, Gainesville, Florida.

Mellon, M. W., Whiteside, S. P., & Friedrich, W. N. (2006). The relevance of fecal soiling as an indicator of child sexual abuse: A preliminary analysis. *Journal of Developmental and Behavioral Pediatrics, 27*, 25–32.

Meunier, P., Mollard, P., & Marechal, J. M. (1976). Physiopathology of megarectum: The association of megarectum with encopresis. *Gut, 17*, 224–227.

Mikkelson, E. J., & Rapoport, J. L. (1980). Enuresis: Psychopathology, sleep stage, and drug response. *Urological Clinics of North America, 7*, 361–377.

Moffatt, M. E. (1989). Nocturnal enuresis: Psychologic implications of treatment and non-treatment. *Journal of Pediatrics, 114*, 697–704.

Moffatt, M. E. (1997). Nocturnal enuresis: A review of the efficacy of treatments and practical advice for clinicians. *Journal of Developmental and Behavioral Pediatrics, 18*, 49–56.

Moffatt, M. E., Harlos, S., Kirshen, A. J., & Burd, L. (1993). Desmopressin acetate and nocturnal enuresis: How much do we know? *Pediatrics, 92*, 420–425.

Moffat, E. K. (1989). Nocturnal enuresis: Psychologic implications of treatment and non-treatment. *Journal of Pediatrics, 114*, 697–704.

Mowrer, O. H., & Mowrer, W. M. (1938). Enuresis: A method for its study and treatment. *American Journal of Orthopsychiatry, 8*, 436–459.

Muellner, R. S. (1960). Development of urinary control in children. *Journal of the American Medical Association, 172*, 1256–1261.

Muellner, R. S. (1961). Obstacles to the successful treatment of primary enuresis. *Journal of the American Medical Association, 178*, 147–148.

Nelson, R. (1977). Methodological issues in assessment via self-monitoring. In J. D. Norgaard, J. P., Pedersen, E. B., & Djurhuus, J. C. (1985). Diurnal antidiuretic hormone levels in enuretics. *Journal of Urology, 134*, 1029–31.

O'Brien, S., Ross, L. V., & Christophersen, E. R. (1986). Primary encopresis: Evaluation and treatment. *Journal of Applied Behavior Analysis, 19*, 137–145.

Olness, K. (1975). The use of self hypnosis in the treatment of childhood nocturnal enuresis. *Clinical Pediatrics, 14*, 273–279.

Oswald, K., Taylor, A. M., & Treisman, M. (1960). Discriminative responses to stimulation during human sleep. *Brain, 83*, 440–445.

Owens-Stively, J. (1995). *Childhood constipation and soiling: A practical guide for parents and children* (2nd ed.). Minneapolis, MN: Children's Health Care.

Pashankar, D. S., Loening-Baucke, V., & Bishop, W. P. (2003). Safety of Polyethylene Glycol for the treatment of chronic constipation in children. *Archives of Pediatric & Adolescent Medicine: 157*, 661–664.

Partin, J. C., Hamill, S. K., Fischel, J. E., & Partin, J. S. (1992). Painful defecation and fecal soiling in children. *Pediatrics, 89*, 1007–1009.

Pickering, L. K., Bartlett, A. V., & Woodward, W. E. (1986). Acute infectious diarrhea among children in day care: Epidemiology and control. *Review of Infectious Disease, 8*, 539–547

Powell, N. B. (1951). Urinary incontinence in children. *Archives of Pediatrics, 68*, 151–157.

Rauber A., & Maroncelli, R. (1984). Prescribing practices and knowledge of tricyclic anti-depressants among physicians caring for children. *Pediatrics, 73*, 107–109.

Reynolds, C. R., & Kamphaus, R. W. (1992). *Behavior Assessment System for Children: Manual.* Circle Pines, MN: American Guidance.

Richmond, J. B., Eddy, E. J., & Garrard, S. D. (1954). The syndrome of fecal soiling and megacolon. *American Journal of Orthopsychiatry, 24*, 391–401.

Robinson, E. A., Eyberg, S. M., & Ross, A. W. (1980). Inventory of child behavior problems. *Journal of Clinical Child Psychology*, Spring, 22–29

Rockney, R. M., McQuade, W. H., & Days, A. L. (1995). The plain abdominal roentgenogram in the management of encopresis. *Archives of Pediatrics & Adolescent Medicine, 149*, 623–627.

Rockney, R. M., McQuade, W. H., Days, A. L., Linn, H. E., & Alario, A. J. (1996). Encopresis treatment outcome: Long-term follow-up of 45 cases. *Journal of Developmental & Behavioral Pediatrics, 17*, 380–385.

Rolider, A., & Van Houten, R. (1986). Effects of degree of awakening and the criterion for advancing awakening on the treatment of bedwetting. *Education and Treatment of Children, 9,* 135–141.

Rolider, A., Van Houten, & Chlebowski, I. (1984). Effects of a stringent versus lenient awakening procedure on the efficacy of the dry bed procedure. *Child and Family Behavior Therapy, 14,* 1–14.

Ronen, T., Wozner, Y., & Rahav, G. (1992). Cognitive intervention in enuresis. *Child and Family Behavior Therapy, 14,* 1–14.

Ruckstuhl, L. E. (2003). Evaluation of the vibrating urine alarm: A study of effectiveness, social validity, and path to continence for enuretic children. *Dissertation Abstracts International: Section B: The Sciences and Engineering, 64* (5B), 2376. (UMI No. AAI309087).

Rutter, M., Tizard, J., & Whitmore, K. (1970). *Education, health, and behavior.* London: Longmans.

Safder, S., Rewalt, M., & Elitsur, Y. (2006). Digital rectal examination and the primary-care physician: A lost art? *Clinical Pediatrics, 45,* 411–414.

Schaefer, C. E. (1995). *Childhood enuresis and encopresis.* Lanham, MD: Jason Aronson.

Scharf, M. B., & Jennings, S. W. (1988). Childhood enuresis: Relationship to sleep, etiology, evaluation, and treatment. *Annals of Behavioral Medicine, 10,* 113–120.

Shreeram, S., He, J., Kalaydjian, A., Brothers, S., & Merikangas, K. (2009). Prevalence of enuresis and its association with attention-deficit/hyperactivity disorder among US children: Results from a nationally representative study. *Journal of the American Academy of Child and Adolescent Psychiatry, 48,* 35–41.

Schneider, M. S., King, L. R., & Surwitt, R. S. (1994). Kegel exercises and childhood incontinence: A new role for an old treatment. *Journal of Pediatrics, 124,* 91–92.

Schonwald, A., Sherritt, L., Stadtler, A., & Bridgemohan, C. (2004). Factors associated with difficult toilet training. *Pediatrics, 113,* 1753–1757.

Schonwald, A. D., & Sheldon, G. G. (2006). *The pocket idiot's guide to potty training problems.* Indianapolis, IN: Penguin Group.

Schonwald, A. D., & Rappaport, L. A. (2008). Elimination conditions. In M. L. Wolraich, D. D. Drotar, P. H. Dworkin, & E. C. Perrin (Eds), *Developmental-behavioral pediatrics* (pp. 791–04). Philadelphia, PA: Mosby.

Schaefer, C. E. (1995). *Childhood enuresis and encopresis.* Lanham, MD: Jason Aronson.

Shaffer, D., Gardner, A., & Hedge, B. (1984). Behavior and bladder disturbance of enuretic children: A rational classification of a common disorder. *Developmental Medicine & Child Neurology, 26,* 781–792.

Sigelman, C. K., & Begley, N. L. (1987). The early development of reactions to peers with controllable and uncontrollable problems. *Journal of Pediatric Psychology, 12,* 99–114.

Slavkin, M. L., & Shohov (2004). Predictive validity of the ego triad: The myth of enuresis, firesetting, and cruelty to animals. In S. P. Shohov (Ed.), *Advances in psychology research, Vol. 31* (pp. 199–206). Hauppage, NY: Nova Science Publishers.

Society for Pediatric Gastroenterology, Hepatology, and Nutrition (2006). Clinical Practice Guideline: Evaluation and treatment of constipation in infants and children: Recommendations of the North American Society for Pediatric Gastroenterology, Hepatology and Nutrition. *Journal of Pediatric Gastroentology and Nutrition, 43,* e1–e13.

Sperling, M. (1994). *The major neuroses & behavior disorders in children.* Northvale, NJ: Aronoson.

Stanton, H. (1979). Short term treatment of enuresis. *American Journal of Clinical Hypnosis, 22,* 103–107.

Starfield, B. (1967). Functional bladder capacity in enuretic and nonenuretic children. *Journal of Pediatrics, 70,* 777–782.

Starfield, B., & Mellits, E. D. (1968). Increases in functional bladder capacity and improvements in enuresis. *Journal of Pediatrics, 72,* 483–487.

Stark, L. J. (2000). Commentary: Treatment of encopresis: Where do we go from here? *Journal of Pediatric Psychology, 25,* 255–256.

Stark, L. J., Opipari, L. C., Donaldson, D. L., Danovsky, M. B., Rasile, D. A., & Del Santo, A. F. (1997). Evaluation of a standard protocol for retentive encopresis: A replication. *Journal of Pediatric Psychology, 22*, 619–633.

Stark, L. J., Owens-Stively, J., Spirito, A., Lewis, A., & Guevremont, D. (1990). Group behavioral treatment of retentive encopresis. *Journal of Pediatric Psychology, 15*, 659–671.

Sutphen, J. L., Borowitz, S. M., Hutchison, R. L., & Cox, D. J. (1995). Long-term follow-up of medically treated childhood constipation. *Clinical Pediatrics, 34*, 576–580.

Tarbox, R., Williams, L., & Friman, P.C. (2004). Extended diaper wearing: Effects on continence in and out of the diaper. *Journal of Applied Behavior Analysis, 37*, 97–101.

Taubman, B. (1997). Toilet training and toileting refusal for stool only: A prospective study. *Pediatrics, 99*, 54–58.

Turner, R., Young, G., & Rachman, S. (1970). Treatment of nocturnal enuresis by conditioning techniques. *Behavior Research & Therapy, 8*, 367–381.

Troup, C. W., & Hodgson, N. B. (1971). Nocturnal functional bladder capacity in enuretic children. *Journal of Urology, 105* 129–132.

US Food and Drug Administration. (2007). Desmopressin Acetate (marketed as DDAVP Nasal Spray, DDAVP Rhinal Tube, DDAVP, DDVP, Minirin, and Stimate Nasal Spray). Retrieved February 21, 2009 from, http://www.fda.gov/Safety/MedWatch/SafetyInformation/SafetyAlertsforHumanMedicalProducts/ucm079928.htm

Van Dijk, M., Bongers, M. E. J., deVries, G., Grootenhuis, M. A., Last, B. F., & Benninga, M. A. (2008). *Pediatrics, 121*, e1334–e1341.

Van Laecke, E., Wille, S., Vande Walle, J., Raes, A., Renson, C., Peeren, F., & Hoebeke, P. (2006). The daytime alarm: A useful device for the treatment of children with daytime incontinence. *The Journal of Urology, 176*, 325–327.

Van Tijen, N. M., Messer, A. P., & Namdar, Z. (1998). Perceived stress of nocturnal enuresis in childhood. *British Journal of Urology, 81* (Suppl. 3), 98–99.

Verhulst, F. C., van der Lee, J. H., Akkeruis, G. W., Sanders-Woudstra, J. A. R., Timmer, F. C., & Donkhorst, I. D. (1985). The prevalence of nocturnal enuresis: Do DSM-III criteria need to be changed? A brief research report. *Journal of Child Psychology and Psychiatry, 26*, 989–993.

Vincent, S. A. (1974). Mechanical, electrical and other aspects of enuresis. In J. H. Johnston, & W. Goodwin (Eds.), *Reviews in Pediatric Urology* (pp. 280–313). New York: Elsevier.

Vogel, W., Young, M., & Primack W. (1996). A survey of physician use of treatment methods for functional enuresis. *Journal of Developmental Behavioral Pediatrics, 17*, 90–3.

Weaver, L.T., & Steiner, H. (1984). The bowel habits of young children. *Archives of Disease in Childhood, 59*, 649–652.

Weinstock, L. B., & Clouse, R. E. (1987). A focused overview of gastrointestinal physiology. *Annals of Behavioral Medicine, 9*, 3–6.

Whelan, J. P., & Houts, A. C. (1990). Effects of a waking schedule on primary enuretic children treated with full spectrum home training. *Health Psychology, 9*, 164–176.

Williams C. L., Bollella, M., & Wynder, E. L. (1995). A new recommendation for dietary fiber in childhood. *Pediatrics, 96*, 985–988.

Wright, L. (1975). Outcome of a standardized program for treating psychogenic encopresis. *Professional Psychology, 6*, 453–456.

Wright, L., & Walker, C. E. (1976). Behavioral treatment of encopresis. *Clinical Psychologist, 29*, 16–19.

Zung, W. W., & Wilson, W. P. (1961). Responses to auditory stimulation during sleep. *Archives of General Psychiatry, 4*, 548–552.

Appendices: Tools and Resources

The following tools and resources are found in the appendices:

Appendix 1: Dietary Fiber Content of Foods
Appendix 2: Bowel Symptom Rating Sheet
Appendix 3: Representative Child and Parent Handout for Alarm Treatment
Appendix 4: Websites

Appendix 1: Dietary Fiber Content of Foods

The following table serves to help you obtain the recommended amount of dietary fiber in your child's diet. Many new high-fiber foods are coming on the market each week. Watch for them! Check food labels for actual grams of dietary fiber per serving.

Food	Serving size	Dietary fiber (g)	Food	Serving size	Dietary fiber (g)
Breads and crackers			**Cereals**		
Fiberich bread™	1 slice	3.2	Fiber One™	1 cup	24.0
Seven-grain bead	1 slice	3.0	100% bran cereal	1 cup	20.0
High bran "health bread"	1 slice	3.0	Corn Bran™	1 cup	8.0
Cornbread	1 square (1 1/2")	3.0	Cracklin' Oat Bran™	1 cup	8.0
100% whole wheat bread	1 slice	2.4	Fruit n' Fiber™	1 cup	8.0
Cracked wheat bread	1 slice	2.1	Granola	1 cup	7.0
Whole wheat crackers	6	2.0	Shredded Wheat and Bran™	1 cup	6.0
Rye crackers	3	2.0	Raisin Nut Bran™	1 cup	6.0
Whole wheat croutons	1/4 cup	1.5	Raisin Bran™	1 cup	4.0
Rye bread	1 slice	1.2	Oatmeal, cooked	3/4 cup	3.0
White bread	1 slice	0.8	Cheerios™	1 cup	1.8
Flours			**Nuts and Seeds**		
Bran (millers)	1 cup	48.0	Peanuts	1/2 cup	5.5
Cornmeal, stoneground	1 cup	16.5	Almonds	10	3.6
100% whole wheat	1 cup	14.4	Soy nuts	2 Tbsp	3.0
100% rye	1 cup	14.4	Sunflower seeds	2Tbsp	3.0
Rolled oats	1 cup	12.0	Walnuts	1/2 cup	3.0
All-purpose white flour	1 cup	1.6	Peanut butter	2 Tbsp	2.0
Fruits			**Vegetables**		
Figs, dried	2	8.0	Baked beans	1 cup	18.6
Apricots, dried	8	7.8	Peas	1 cup	11.3
Dates, dried	10	7.0	Corn	1 cup	9.3
Raisins	1/2 cup	5.4	Broccoli	2 spears	7.0
Prunes, dried	4	5.2	Yams, baked with skin	1 medium	6.8
Orange	1 medium	4.5	Green beans	1 cup	3.5
Banana	1 medium	4.0	Spinach	1 cup	3.5
Apple, with peel	1 medium	3.3	Carrots	1 cup	3.2
Strawberries	1 cup	3.3	Potatoes, baked with skin	1 medium	3.0
Pear	1 medium	3.1	Tomato	1 medium	3.0
Cantaloupe	1/4 medium	2.5	Cabbage, shredded	1 cup	1.9
Plums	2	2.5	Lettuce	1 cup	0.8
Apricots	3	2.4	Celery	1 stalk	0.7

Adapted with permission from Owens-Stively, J. (1995). *Childhood constipation and soiling: A practical guide for parents and children* (2nd ed.). Minneapolis, MN: Children's Health Care.

Appendix 2: Bowel Symptom Rating Sheet

	Amount of medicatioon	# of supp.	# of enemas	# of soilings	# BM's in toilet	Size/consistency	# grams of fiber	Amt. of liquids	Type of activity	Time reward	Comments
1											
2											
3											
4											
5											
6											
7											
8											
9											
10											
11											
12											
13											
14											
15											
16											
17											
18											
19											
20											
21											
22											
23											
24											
25											
26											
27											
28											
29											
30											
31											

KEY: Medication: # of tablespoons/g
        Size/Consistency: Approx. no. of cups; H = hard, S = soft, D = diarrhea
        Amt. of liquids: No. of glasses of water or juice per day
        Activity: 3 = much activity, 2 = moderate activity, 1 = little activity
        Time: Indicates how parent spent reward time with child

Appendix 3: Representative Child and Parent Handout for Alarm Treatment

Your bedwetting alarm will help you to stop wetting the bed. The alarm wakes you up when you start to wet so that you can either stop and go back to sleep or get up and go to the bathroom. The fastest and best way to stop having accidents is to use the alarm every night. Follow these steps:

1. Hook up the alarm by yourself. If you need help, ask your mom or dad, but eventually learn to do it on your own. To get better at using it, practice attaching it to your clothes. Then make it go off and practice going to the bathroom, just like you would at night.
2. Give yourself a pep talk just before bed. Tell yourself you are going to beat the alarm. Then imagine waking up before when you first have the urge to go to the bathroom and really holding it or getting up very quickly and going to the bathroom.
3. If the alarm does go off, try to wake up as quickly as you can, turn it off, and go immediately to the bathroom. If you are having trouble waking up, ask your mom or dad to help you.
4. When you go back to bed, put on clean underwear and pajamas and put clean sheets on your bed.
5. If you are keeping a record, write:
   a. **Dry**: The alarm did not go off
   b. **A little wet**: You got up right after the alarm went off and were a little wet
   c. **Very wet**: You got up right after the alarm went off and were very wet.
   d. **Wet, did not wake up:** You woke in the morning wet.

The alarm is a tool to help your child learn to stop wetting the bed. It rarely works right away, so be prepared for many nights of practice. The alarm will go off immediately after your child starts wetting. Children are likely to sleep through the alarm initially, so you will probably have to help them wake up. This is difficult but very important.

When the alarm goes off, quickly go to your child's room, wake him or her fully, take the child and have him or her eliminate fully in the toilet. Afterwards, help him or her change sheets and pajamas and go back to bed and sleep.

Encourage your child using the alarm *every night*. Your interest in this will increase their chances at a quick success. You and your child will need patience, however: Some children respond quickly, even within the first few weeks whereas others may require many months of training. But most are fully dry within 12 weeks of continuous practice. We recommend your child using the alarm for at least 12 weeks or until he or she has been dry for at least 4 weeks.

Adapted from: The Children's Mercy Hospital (2009). *Care card: "How to use your bedwetting alarm"*.

From: E. R. Christophersen & P. C. Friman: *Elimination Disorders in Children and Adolescents*   © 2010 Hogrefe Publishing

Appendix 4: Websites

- For a variety of toilet training accessories:
  http://www.pottytrainingconcepts.com

- For more information on the Toilet Training School at the Children's Hospital in Boston, MA:
  http://www.childrenshospital.org/az/Site1755/mainpageS1755P0.html

- University of Virginia Health Sciences Center website:
  http://www.hsc.virginia.edu/internet/pediatrics/tutorials/constipation/encopresis.cfm

- The Bedwetting Store:
  http://www.bedwettingstore.com

- Bedwetting facts:
  http://www.aacap.org/cs/root/facts_for_families/bedwetting

- Bedwetting general information:
  http://en.wikipedia.org/wiki/Bedwetting

- Bedwetting and soiling information and treatment:
  http://www.soilingsolutions.com/drybed.htm

- Daytime wetting general information:
  http://www.drspock.com/article/0,1510,5712,00.html

- General information and products for all aspects of child incontinence:
  http://www.pottymd.com

- Family doctor, soiling:
  http://familydoctor.org/online/famdocen/home/children/parents/toilet/166.html